Recent Research in Restorative Dental Materials

Recent Research in Restorative Dental Materials

Guest Editors

Leszek Szalewski
Ingrid K. Różyło-Kalinowska

MDPI

Basel • Beijing • Wuhan • Barcelona • Belgrade • Novi Sad • Cluj • Manchester

Guest Editors
Leszek Szalewski
Digital Dentistry Lab
Department of Dental and
Maxillofacial Radiodiagnostics
Medical University of Lublin
Lublin
Poland

Ingrid K. Różyło-Kalinowska
Department of Dental and
Maxillofacial Radiodiagnostics
Medical University of Lublin
Lublin
Poland

Editorial Office
MDPI AG
Grosspeteranlage 5
4052 Basel, Switzerland

This is a reprint of the Special Issue, published open access by the journal *Materials* (ISSN 1996-1944), freely accessible at: https://www.mdpi.com/journal/materials/special_issues/6410366W6D.

For citation purposes, cite each article independently as indicated on the article page online and as indicated below:

Lastname, A.A.; Lastname, B.B. Article Title. *Journal Name* **Year**, *Volume Number*, Page Range.

ISBN 978-3-7258-6554-3 (Hbk)
ISBN 978-3-7258-6555-0 (PDF)
https://doi.org/10.3390/books978-3-7258-6555-0

Contents

About the Editors

Leszek Szalewski

Leszek Szalewski is a dentist and academic researcher specializing in restorative dentistry and dental materials science. He has extensive clinical experience combining conservative dentistry, prosthodontics, and endodontics with academic and research activities. His scientific interests focus on contemporary restorative materials, digital dentistry, dental photography, and the evaluation of material properties and clinical performance. He is actively involved in undergraduate and postgraduate education and has contributed to numerous scientific publications and conference presentations. His work emphasizes the integration of modern material science with evidence-based clinical practice in restorative dentistry.

Ingrid K. Różyło-Kalinowska

Ingrid K. Różyło-Kalinowska is a full professor in medical sciences and an experienced academic teacher and researcher. Her scientific work focuses on dental radiology, imaging diagnostics, and the application of modern technologies in dentistry. She has authored and co-authored numerous peer-reviewed scientific publications and has actively participated in national and international research projects. Professor Różyło-Kalinowska is deeply engaged in undergraduate and postgraduate education and has played a significant role in advancing evidence-based approaches in dental diagnostics and clinical practice.

Preface

This Reprint brings together a carefully selected collection of scientific contributions dedicated to recent advances in restorative dental materials. Its scope encompasses contemporary material solutions used in restorative dentistry, with a particular emphasis on their composition, properties, clinical performance, and interaction with the oral environment. This Reprint therefore reflects the dynamic development of materials science as applied to dentistry, spanning experimental investigations, translational research, and clinically oriented studies.

The primary aim of this Reprint is to provide a coherent and up-to-date overview of how modern restorative materials are evolving in response to increasing clinical demands, technological progress, and expectations for long-term treatment success. Advances in composite materials, ceramics, glass-ionomer systems, and hybrid structures are presented alongside innovative fabrication techniques and digital workflows that are reshaping everyday clinical practice. Collectively, these works illustrate how material selection and handling protocols directly influence functional, biological, and esthetic outcomes.

The motivation for preparing this Reprint arises from the growing need to integrate fundamental materials research with evidence-based clinical dentistry. Rapid innovation, while beneficial, also introduces challenges related to durability, predictability, and biological compatibility. By assembling contributions from diverse research groups, this Reprint aims to foster critical reflection, encourage interdisciplinary collaboration, and support informed decision-making in both research and clinical settings.

This Reprint is aimed at dental researchers, material scientists, clinicians, educators, and postgraduate students who seek a deeper understanding of current trends and future directions in restorative dental materials. It is intended to serve not only as a reference summarizing recent progress but also as a stimulus for further investigation and innovation in this continually evolving field.

The Guest Editors hope that this Reprint will contribute meaningfully to the advancement of restorative dentistry by bridging scientific insight and clinical relevance and by highlighting the importance of rigorous evaluation of materials used in everyday patient care.

Leszek Szalewski and Ingrid K. Różyło-Kalinowska
Guest Editors

materials

MDPI

Article

Influence of Low pH on the Microhardness and Roughness Surface of Dental Composite—A Preliminary Study

Leszek Szalewski [1,*], Dorota Wójcik [2], Monika Sowa [3], Vladyslav Vivcharenko [4] and Krzysztof Pałka [3]

1 Digital Dentistry Lab, Department of Dental and Maxillofacial Radiodiagnostics, Medical University of Lublin, 20-059 Lublin, Poland
2 Department of Dental Prosthetics, Medical University of Lublin, 20-059 Lublin, Poland; dorota.wojcik@umlub.pl
3 Deptartment of Materials Engineering, Lublin University of Technology, 20-618 Lublin, Poland; d577@pollub.edu.pl (M.S.); k.palka@pollub.pl (K.P.)
4 Department of Tissue Engineering & Regenerative Medicine, Medical University of Lublin, 20-059 Lublin, Poland
* Correspondence: leszek.szalewski@umlub.pl; Tel.: +48-508-216-949

Abstract: Dental composites are gaining great popularity in restorative dentistry because of their aesthetic appeal and capacity to replicate the natural color of teeth. Nevertheless, their lifespan and durability rely on various factors, such as the polishing technique and the environmental conditions they are exposed to. The study aimed to assess the influence of the method of final polishing of dental composite on the surface roughness and microhardness of materials also considering the environment of different pHs. Disc-shaped samples (5 mm diameter and 2 mm thickness) have been prepared for microhardness and roughness tests from two dental composites: A2 Clearfil Majesty ES 2 Classic and A2D Clearfil Majesty Premium. One-third of samples were polished with polishing discs, OptiDisc, another one-third of samples were polished with Eve Diacomp Twist rubbers and polishing brush with diamond particles, and rest of the samples were stored without any polishing (the control group). Tested materials were incubated in distilled water or acidic buffer (pH = 2) for 3 weeks at a temperature of 37 °C. No statistically significant differences were found for roughness for the two materials tested after incubation in liquids. A decrease in Vicker microhardness was found for Clearfil Majesty ES 2 Classic after soaking in a low pH liquid, and no such relationship was found for Clearfil Majesty Premium. The improved resistance of these materials to the negative oral environment may result in the longer survival of composite restorations in patients with poor diet or diseases, causing a decrease in oral pH.

Keywords: restorative dentistry; aesthetic dentistry; biomechanics; hardness; microscopy; nano-filled composite; surface degradation

1. Introduction

Dental composites have become increasingly popular in restorative dentistry due to their aesthetic appeal and ability to mimic the natural color of teeth. However, their longevity and durability depend on a range of aspects, including the method of polishing and the environmental conditions they are exposed to [1,2]. The polishing of dental composites is crucial to achieve a smooth and glossy surface, which ensures the proper functioning of the stomatognathic system, reduces the accumulation of plaque, and prevents staining [3]. However, polishing can also affect the surface roughness and, subsequently, the mechanical and chemical properties of restoration [4]. Moreover, exposure to acidic environments can cause the degradation of the resin matrix, leading to the deterioration of mechanical properties, discoloration, and microleakage [5]. Recently, several studies have investigated the effect of different polishing methods and acidic environments on the properties of dental composites [6–10]. These studies have used various techniques to evaluate the surface roughness, microhardness, color stability, and degree of conversion of the composites. Composite materials can be polished with abrasive discs, rubber bands, and brushes, with the addition of polishing pastes. In addition, all these methods can be combined in different configurations. Erosion factors from the diet are also not indifferent to the surface of fillings made of composite materials. Low pH values usually have a negative effect on the surface of the fillings [11,12]. Various test liquids were used in the tests: chemical solutions with a known pH or dietary ingredients— drinks (e.g., Cola, tea, orange juice, etc.).

One of the challenges in comparing the results of these studies is the lack of standardization of the testing protocols, including the polishing methods, the type and duration of exposure to acidic environments, and the techniques used to evaluate the properties of the composites. Differences in the results of different studies may be due to diverse sample preparation methodologies. As demonstrated by Ko et al. in their paper on light beam in composite polymerization tips, composite materials undergo inhomogeneous polymerization during exposure [13]. Therefore, it is extremely important in research work to test a similar surface of each specimen with the indenter of a hardness tester, as the results in the center and on the sides of the same specimen can differ significantly. Also, an increase in the distance between the polymerization lamp tip and the composite has an effect on the mechanical properties of the composite materials (such as microhardness) as shown in their study by Hasanain et al. [14]. Additionally, the elimination of the oxygen inhibition layer as well as the polishing of the composite materials can affect the obtained Vickers microhardness results, as shown in their study by Carrillo-Marcos et al. [15]. Both polishing and elimination of the oxygen inhibition layer result in an increase in Vickers microhardness values and a decrease in surface roughness.

Therefore, it is essential to establish standardized testing protocols to enable reliable and accurate comparisons of the properties of dental composite resins.

The null hypothesis of the current study was that the type of polishing and the incubation environment had no effect on microhardness and surface roughness.

2. Materials and Methods

2.1. Specimens' Preparation

Forty-eight disc-shaped samples (5 mm diameter and 2 mm thickness) have been prepared for microhardness and roughness tests for each material. Specimens were produced using a stainless steel mold placed on a microscope slide to achieve a flat surface. The following nanohybrid composites were used in tests, all of the A2 shade: Clearfil Majesty ES 2 Classic (A2C) (Kuraray Europe GmbH, Hattersheim am Main, Germany) and Clearfil Majesty Premium (A2D) (Kuraray Europe GmbH, Hattersheim am Main, Germany). The choice of materials was dictated by differences in application. During filling corrections, the dentin material (A2D) is sometimes exposed beneath the enamel layer (A2C). It is important to check that the dentin material has the same low pH resistance properties as the enamel layer. Advantageously, both materials have a very similar composition: organic matrix—Bis-GMA, dimethacrylate, and photoinitiator (camphorquinone); inorganic filler (78 wt.%)—silanizated barium glass filler, and pre-polymerized organic filler.

Samples were polymerized using a high-powered LED LCU (Mini LED III Supercharged, Acteon Group, Merignac, France). Samples were cured using 10 s pulse-cure mode (total energy = 20 J/cm^2) without any oxygen inhibition layer protection. After photopolymerization, the specimens were released from the mold. The steel mold blocked the light from the side of the samples, which made it possible to obtain reproducible results. There was no risk of false results due to the lateral polymerization of the sample. Next, the specimens were examined under magnification (3.5×) for the presence of air bubbles, and defective specimens were excluded from the study. All specimens were sandblasted (AirNGo, Acteon Group, Merignac, France) with prophylaxis sand (KaVo PROPHYPearls, KaVo Dental GmbH, Warthausen, Germany) for 10 s to eliminate the oxygen inhibition layer.

2.2. *Study Group*

Two additional groups of samples (N = 8 each) were prepared for polishing and conditioning experiments. One group was polished using a series of OptiDisc polishing discs (KerrDental, Brea, USA) from coarse to medium, fine, and extra-fine grits. The other group was polished using a 2-step polishing system with Eve Diacomp Twist rubbers (EVE Ernst Vetter GmbH, Birkenfeld, Germany) followed by polishing with a brush containing diamond particles (EVE Ernst Vetter GmbH, Germany). The final group served as a control and was left unpolished.

After polishing, all specimen groups were immersed in distilled water at 37 °C for 24 h. Subsequently, each of the three main groups was further divided into two subgroups. One subgroup was incubated in 100 mL of distilled water [16], while the other was incubated in 100 mL of acidic solution (pH = 2) (Alfachem Sp. z o.o., Lublin, Poland) for 3 weeks at 37 °C (Figure 1).

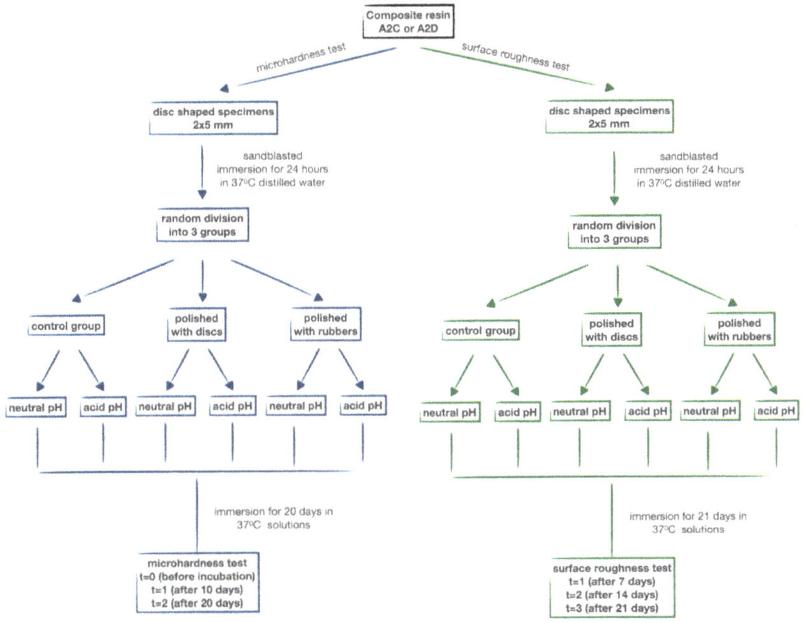

Figure 1. Flow chart of the research process.

The conditioning time in the acidic solution was determined based on guidelines from the study by Gawriołek et al. [17]. According to this protocol, one cup of coffee (150 mL) is assumed to have a 1 min contact time with the oral cavity. Considering a daily consumption of 2 cups (300 mL), each 7 days of sample storage can be correlated to 2 years of material conditioning in the oral environment.

2.3. *Vickers Microhardness Test*

Microhardness measurements were performed using the Vickers method on an FM-800 hardness tester (Future-Tech, Kawasaki-City, Japan) with a load of 0.4905 N, as described in the study by Szalewski et al. [16]. Ten measurements were taken on the photopolymerization side of each sample. The measurements were conducted at three time points: T0 (before incubation), T1 (after 10 days of incubation in the test solution), and T2 (after 20 days of incubation).

2.4. Roughness Test

Surface roughness of the specimens was assessed using an Olympus LEXT OLS5100 3D laser scanning microscope (Olympus Corporation, Tokyo, Japan). Due to the directional nature of the machined surfaces, roughness measurements were conducted using a surface method with the laser microscope. Consistent with the microhardness measurements, the same photopolymerization side of each sample was utilized for these tests. The Sa parameter (arithmetical mean height) was measured four times per sample. Measurements were taken at three time points: T1 (after 7 days of incubation in the test solution), T2 (after 14 days), and T3 (after 21 days).

2.5. Scanning Electron Microscopy (SEM)

The surface morphology of the samples was examined using scanning electron microscopy (SEM). SEM observations were conducted with a Nova NanoSEM 450 (FEI, Eindhoven, The Netherlands) operating in the low-vacuum mode with an accelerating voltage of 5 kV.

2.6. Statistical Methods

Hypotheses related to the differences between the mean values of the Vickers microhardness obtained for incubation solution types and the time of incubation and the polishing protocol were verified by mixed-model ANOVA assumptions analysis, followed by mixed-model ANOVA and post hoc tests. The hypotheses were verified using the significance level of $p = 0.05$. Mean values and standard deviations were calculated. In the first step, the normality of the distribution was analyzed using the Shapiro–Wilk's test, along with the analysis of skewness and kurtosis. In addition, Levene's test was included in the analyses to assess the homogeneity of the variance.

Hypotheses related to the differences between the mean values of the roughness test obtained for incubation solution types and the time of incubation were verified by mixed-model ANOVA assumptions analysis, followed by mixed-model ANOVA and post hoc tests. The hypotheses were verified using the significance level of $p = 0.05$. Mean values and standard deviations were calculated. In the first step, the normality of the distribution was analyzed using the Shapiro–Wilk test, along with the analysis of skewness and kurtosis. In addition, Levene's test was included in the analyses to assess the homogeneity of the variance. The analyses were conducted using the IBM SPSS Statistics 28 software (International Business Machines Corporation, New York, NY, USA).

3. Results

3.1. Vickers Microhardness Test

The results of the microhardness measurements are shown in Figures 2 and 3. Normality tests of the distribution indicate that the normality of the distribution is met in each measurement and soaking method. The assumption of sphericity was met (Mauchly's W = 0.604, $p = 0.469$). An analysis of variance was performed in a mixed scheme, where the within-subject factors were Vickers microhardness before soaking, after 10 days, and after 20 days of induction, the between-subject variables, and the type of fluid in which the samples were soaked. The analysis did not detect significant differences between measurements for the A2D composite; on the other hand, for the A2C composite, significant differences were found between measurements, and the main effect of measurement was statistically significant, $F(2,8) = 10.778$, $p = 0.005$, $\eta^2 = 0.729$. Bonferroni post hoc tests did not show statistically significant differences between measurements for the two materials. Also, the type of polishing had no statistically significant effect on the Vickers microhardness of the composite before and after incubation in the different pH solutions.

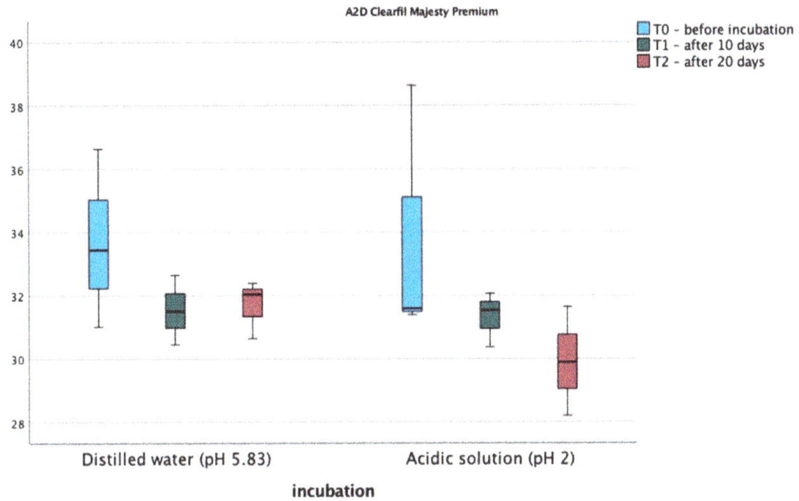

Figure 2. Average Vickers microhardness values for A2D material.

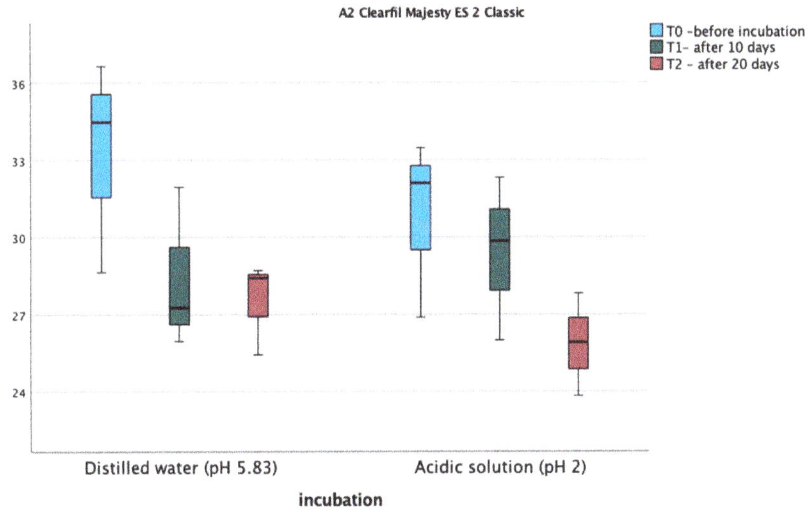

Figure 3. Average Vickers microhardness values for A2C material.

3.2. Roughness Test

Figures 4 and 5 show the average roughness values for the tested materials. The assumption of sphericity was met (Mauchly's W = 0.716, $p = 0.606$). An analysis of variance was performed in a mixed design scheme, where the within-subject factors were roughness after 1 week, 2 weeks, and 3 weeks of soaking, the between-subject variables, and the type of fluid in which the sample was soaked. Bonferroni post hoc tests for both materials showed no statistically significant differences between measurements. Also, the type of polishing had no statistically significant effect on the roughness of the composite before and after incubation in the different pH solutions.

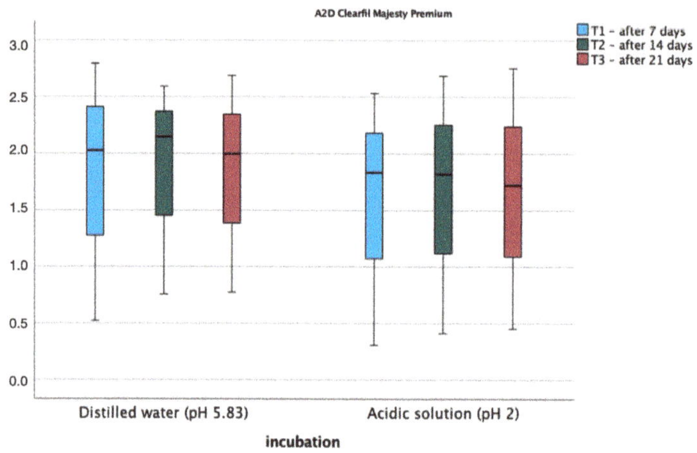

Figure 4. Average roughness values for A2D material.

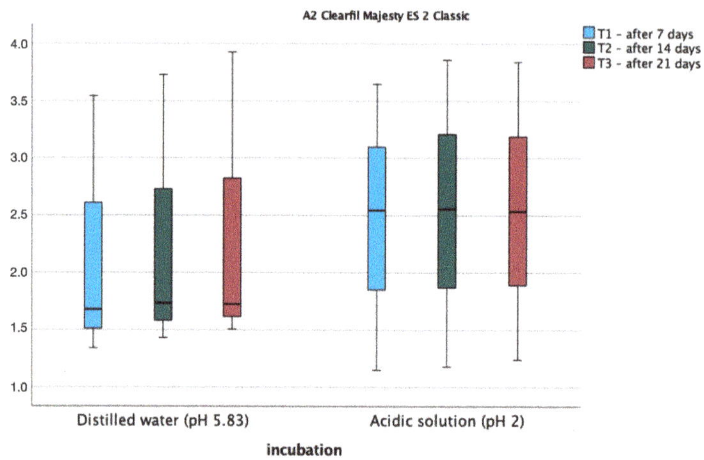

Figure 5. Average roughness values for A2C material.

3.3. *Scanning Electron Microscopy (SEM)*

The SEM images presented in Figures 6 and 7 reveal distinct differences in the surface morphology of the composite resin materials. The surfaces of the untreated, unpolished specimens exhibited the smoothest appearance (Figures 6a and 7a). When polishing rubbers were used, the SEM images showed evidence of composite resin filler loss on the surface (Figures 6d and 7d). This suggests that the polishing process with rubbers resulted in the removal of some of the resin filler particles. In the case of abrasive discs, the directionality of the polishing process is visible on the surface (Figures 6g and 7g). This is likely due to the standardized unidirectional polishing protocol used to maintain consistency across the samples. After soaking the specimens in both neutral pH and acidic pH solutions, the degradation of the matte surface was observed (Figures 6e,f,h,i and 7e,f,h,i). The changes were more pronounced in the acidic pH conditions, where eroded areas of the surface could be seen. Importantly, no cracks or mechanical damage were detected on the surfaces of the samples during the polishing procedures. This indicates that the polishing protocols employed did not result in any visible structural damage to the composite resin materials.

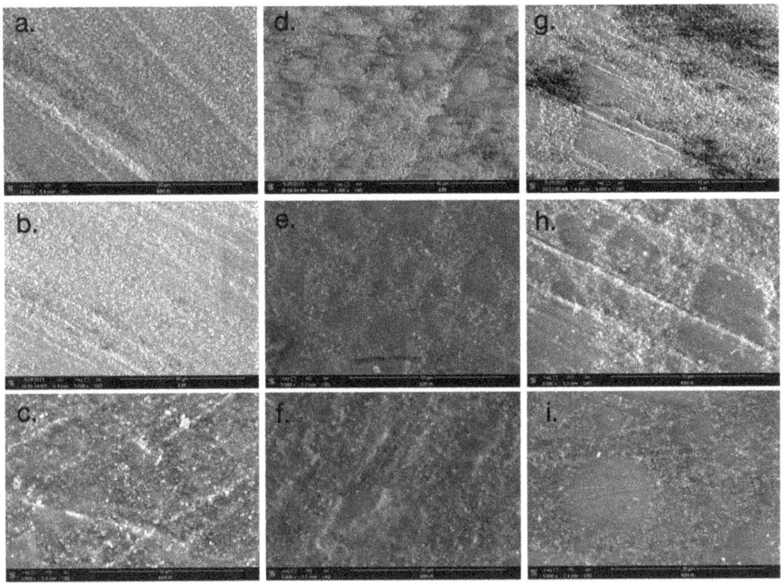

Figure 6. SEM images of A2C composite (magnification: ×5000): (**a**) A2C t = 0; (**b**) A2C t = 21 days, pH neutral; (**c**) A2C t = 21 days, pH acidic; (**d**) A2C_G t = 0; (**e**) A2C_G t = 21 days, pH neutral; (**f**) A2C_G t = 21 days, pH acidic; (**g**) A2C_K t = 0; (**h**) A2C_K t = 21 days, pH neutral; and (**i**) A2C_K t = 21 days, pH acidic.

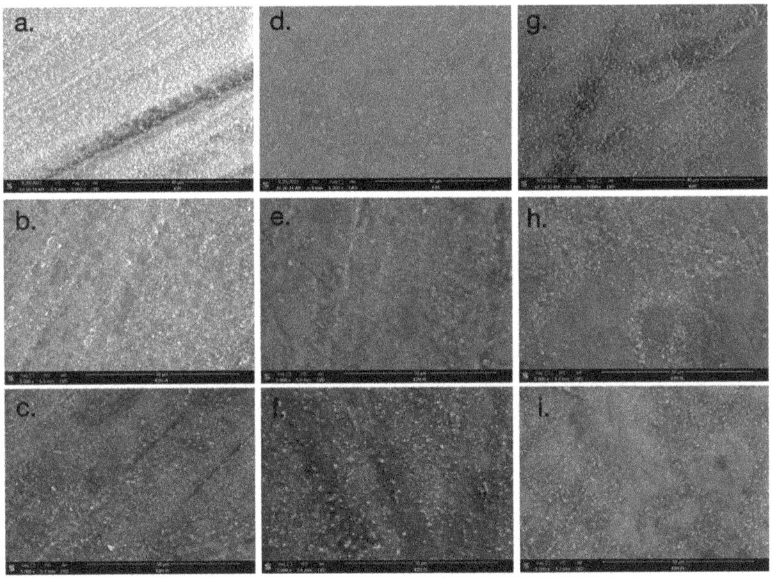

Figure 7. SEM images of A2D composite (magnification: ×5000): (**a**) A2D t = 0; (**b**) A2D t = 21 days, pH neutral; (**c**) A2D t = 21 days, pH acidic; (**d**) A2D_G t = 0; (**e**) A2D_G t = 21 days, pH neutral; (**f**) A2D_G t = 21 days, pH acidic; (**g**) A2D_K t = 0; (**h**) A2D_K t = 21 days, pH neutral; and (**i**) A2D_K t = 21 days, pH acidic.

4. Discussion

The null hypothesis was confirmed in the case of the A2D material for both tested parameters, and in the case of the A2C material, the roughness is not affected by the tested factors, but the Vickers microhardness of the material decreases after a 3-week incubation at low pH.

A decrease in oral pH can be attributed to various factors, including dietary abnormalities, impaired mineral balance, or systemic diseases. This acidic environment can adversely affect the mechanical and functional properties of dental restorative materials. The maintenance of excellent mechanical properties and resistance to environmental changes in the oral cavity is crucial for composite materials used in dentistry. Over the years, manufacturers have refined both the application and polymerization procedures of composite materials, as well as their composition, to achieve optimal properties for dental restorations. In a study by Kumari et al., none of the tested composite materials exhibited changes in Vickers microhardness after exposure to citric acid (low pH) compared to storage in neutral pH (air) [18]. Our research corroborates these findings for the A2D material; however, the A2C material demonstrated a decrease in Vickers microhardness. Hamdy et al. similarly reported no statistically significant difference in the Vickers microhardness of tested composite materials after immersion in mouthwashes [19], which partially aligns with our results. It should be noted, however, that their methodology involved only a 24 h immersion period, which may be insufficient to observe significant changes. Kumari et al.'s study also revealed varying initial microhardness values among the tested materials, ranging from 28.35 to 96.76 HV. Contrasting results were obtained by Barve et al., who observed a statistically significant reduction in Vickers microhardness values for Filtek Z250 material stored in Cola (low pH) after a 15-day immersion period compared to the control sample (distilled water) [20]. Unal et al. also noted a decrease in the Vickers microhardness of composite materials after 14 days of exposure to gastric acid, simulating conditions associated with diseases causing frequent vomiting, such as bulimia [21]. In their study, the extent of Vickers microhardness reduction varied depending on the material tested, ranging from 35% (Beautifil II) to 16% (Filtek Z550). Similarly, Vecek et al. reported a reduction in the Vickers microhardness of composite materials by 8–28% after a 30-day incubation in a green smoothie, which aligns with our findings for the A2C material [22]. Additionally, composite materials in the oral cavity are exposed to other factors, such as tooth-whitening products. Fernandes et al. demonstrated that tooth-whitening formulations based on 35% hydrogen peroxide or 16% carbamide peroxide can cause up to a 10% decrease in Knoop microhardness [23].

The effects of low pH environments on the surface roughness of dental composite materials have been examined in several studies, yielding mixed results. Kumari et al. observed that exposure to a low pH citric acid solution led to a statistically significant decrease in surface roughness for half of the tested composite materials (Tetric Evo Ceram and Filtek Z350), while the remaining materials (Clearfil Majesty and EverX) showed no change in roughness [18]. In contrast, Camilotti et al. reported an increase in roughness after just 30 days of immersion in low pH solutions (pH = 2.73, 2.74, 3.58), with further increases noted over extended periods of 90 and 180 days [24]. Tavangara et al. conducted a study on three different composite materials polished with Soflex discs and found that soaking in low pH liquids (pH = 2.47 for Coke and pH = 5.41 for coffee) resulted in an increase in roughness compared to a control group soaked in distilled water [25]. These findings diverge from those of the current study, which found no statistically significant difference in surface roughness after soaking the composite materials in an acidic liquid. The research by Vaidya et al. demonstrated that liquid composite materials exhibit increased roughness when exposed to acidic beverages, including energy drinks and alcoholic beverages [26]. However, bulk-fill composite materials showed resilience to short-term acid exposure, with no significant roughness changes observed after a 60 min immersion combined with brushing simulation [10]. This suggests that newer composite materials may possess enhanced acid resistance, although mechanical hygiene practices continue to significantly influence surface characteristics. Lepri and Palma-Dibb's study further nuanced these findings, indicating that acid immersion alone may not significantly alter roughness compared to neutral pH conditions [27]. However, the combination of acid exposure and brushing resulted in statistically significant increases in roughness. These results underscore the complex interplay between environmental factors and mechanical stress in determining the surface properties of dental composites. The divergent outcomes across studies highlight the need for standardized methodologies and consideration of material-specific responses when evaluating the effects of acidic environments on dental composites.

The roughness of composite materials significantly influences their longevity in the patient's mouth. Guo et al. demonstrated that materials with greater initial roughness tend to wear out more quickly [8]. The process is further accelerated when these materials are soaked in low pH fluids (pH = 5.5) compared to a control group (pH = 7.05). This acceleration may be attributed to the loss of ceramic particles during polishing, as observed in SEM studies. Our study also noted a clear loss of filler particles post-polishing with rubbers or polishing discs, an effect that intensifies after exposure to acidic pH. The literature reports similar findings, indicating an increase in roughness following the finishing of composite materials with rotary tools [7]. Notably, composites treated with Enchance rubbers exhibited higher surface roughness compared to those polished with Soflex discs similar to our results. SEM images from our study revealed the dissolution of the organic matrix in composite materials after aging in both neutral and acidic solutions. Consequently, composites with a higher filler content are more resistant to low pH environments. This observation is corroborated by Sideridou et al., who reported that the degradation of composite surfaces occurs due to the hydrolysis of the organic matrix and the release of filler particles [28]. This degradation leads to a decrease in Vickers microhardness and an increase in material roughness.

Based on the obtained results, it can be concluded that the proper finishing of composite materials yields surfaces with adequate smoothness, which remain largely unaffected by low pH dietary conditions. Nevertheless, patients should be advised that the consumption of acidic foods may lead to material degradation, manifesting as decreased Vickers microhardness. This degradation could potentially result in compromised marginal integrity, discoloration, cracking, and ultimately necessitate restoration replacement. To enhance the mechanical properties of composite restorations, such as Vickers microhardness and flexural strength, dental practitioners should consider employing extended polymerization times for the final layer or utilizing polymerization units with higher energy output [29,30]. These measures may contribute to improved longevity and performance of composite restorations in the oral environment.

5. Conclusions

The study found a decrease in Vickers microhardness for one test material (Clearfil Majesty Es-2) after immersion in a low pH liquid (pH = 2) compared to a neutral solution (pH = 5.83). However, there was no significant correlation between the soaked fluid and the roughness of the composite materials. These results may suggest an improvement in the mechanical properties of the new composite materials, as exemplified by Clearfil Majesty Es-2 and Clearfil Majesty Premium. The enhanced resistance of these materials to the hostile oral environment may lead to longer survival of composite restorations in patients with poor dietary habits or diseases, causing a decrease in oral pH.

Author Contributions: Conceptualization, L.S. and K.P.; methodology, K.P. and M.S.; software, D.W. and V.V.; validation, L.S., D.W. and K.P.; formal analysis, K.P. and M.S.; investigation, M.S. and V.V.; resources, L.S.; data curation, D.W. and K.P.; writing—original draft preparation, L.S. and K.P.; writing—review and editing, D.W., M.S. and V.V.; visualization, D.W. and K.P.; supervision, L.S. and K.P.; project administration, L.S. All authors have read and agreed to the published version of the manuscript.

Funding: This research received no external funding.

Institutional Review Board Statement: Not applicable.

Informed Consent Statement: Not applicable.

Data Availability Statement: Data are contained within the article.

Conflicts of Interest: The authors declare no conflicts of interest.

References

1. Dionysopoulos, D.; Gerasimidou, O. Wear of contemporary dental composite resin restorations: A literature review. *Restor. Dent. Endod.* **2021**, *46*, e18. [CrossRef] [PubMed] [PubMed Central]
2. Elfakhri, F.; Alkahtani, R.; Li, C.; Khaliq, J. Influence of filler characteristics on the performance of dental composites: A comprehensive review. *Ceram. Int.* **2022**, *48*, 27280–27294. [CrossRef]
3. Vishwanath, S.; Kadandale, S.; Kumarappan, S.K.; Ramachandran, A.; Unnikrishnan, M.; Nagesh, H.M. Finishing and Polishing of Composite Restoration: Assessment of Knowledge, Attitude and Practice Among Various Dental Professionals in India. *Cureus* **2022**, *14*, e20887. [CrossRef] [PubMed]
4. Szczepaniak, M.E.; Krasowski, M.; Bołtacz-Rzepkowska, E. The Effect of Various Polishing Systems on the Surface Roughness of Two Resin Composites—An In Vitro Study. *Coatings* **2022**, *12*, 916. [CrossRef]
5. Da Silva, T.M.; Sales, A.L.L.S.; Pucci, C.R.; Borges, A.B.; Torres, C.R.G. The combined effect of food-simulating solutions, brushing and staining on color stability of composite resins. *Acta Biomater. Odontol. Scand.* **2017**, *3*, 1276838. [CrossRef] [PubMed]
6. Deljoo, Z.; Sadeghi, M.; Azar, M.R.; Bagheri, R. The Effect of Different Polishing Methods and Storage Media on Discoloration of Resin Composites. *J. Dent. Biomater.* **2016**, *3*, 226–232.
7. Valinoti, A.C.; Neves, B.G.; da Silva, E.M.; Maia, L.C. Surface degradation of composite resins by acidic medicines and ph-cycling. *J. Appl. Oral Sci.* **2008**, *16*, 257–265. [CrossRef]
8. Guo, J.; Bing, Z.; Yang, J.; Tsoi, J.K.H.; Wang, Y. Effect of roughness and acidic medium on wear behavior of dental resin composite. *BMC Oral Health* **2022**, *22*, 470. [CrossRef]
9. Münchow, E.A.; Ferreira, A.C.A.; Machado, R.M.M.; Ramos, T.S.; Rodrigues-Junior, S.A.; Zanchi, C.H. Effect of Acidic Solutions on the Surface Degradation of a Micro-Hybrid Composite Resin. *Braz. Dent. J.* **2014**, *25*, 321–326. [CrossRef]
10. Tărăboanță, I.; Buhățel, D.; Brînză Concită, C.A.; Andrian, S.; Nica, I.; Tărăboanță-Gamen, A.C.; Brânzan, R.; Stoleriu, S. Evaluation of the Surface Roughness of Bulk-Fill Composite Resins after Submission to Acidic and Abrasive Aggressions. *Biomedicines* **2022**, *10*, 1008. [CrossRef]
11. Khan, A.A.; Siddiqui, A.Z.; Al-Kheraif, A.A.; Zahid, A.; Divakar, D.D. Effect of different pH solvents on micro-hardness and surface topography of dental nano-composite: An in vitro analysis. *Pak. J. Med. Sci.* **2015**, *31*, 854–859. [CrossRef] [PubMed] [PubMed Central]
12. Singh, T.; Mahalakshmi, V.; Sahu, S.; Chatterjee, S.; Khan, A.M.; Haqh, M.F.; Singh, V. A Comparative Evaluation of the Effect of Different Beverages on Colour Stability and Surface Micromorphology of Nanocomposite Restorative Material. *Cureus* **2023**, *15*, e41905. [CrossRef] [PubMed] [PubMed Central]
13. Ko, H.; Kim, D.; Park, S.-H. Homogeneity of dental curing unit beam profile and its effect on microhardness of dental composites with varying thicknesses. *Dent. Mater.* **2022**, *38*, e231–e243. [CrossRef] [PubMed]
14. Hasanain, F.A.; Nassar, H.M.; Ajaj, R.A. Effect of Light Curing Distance on Microhardness Profiles of Bulk-Fill Resin Composites. *Polymers* **2022**, *14*, 528. [CrossRef] [PubMed]
15. Carrillo-Marcos, A.; Salazar-Correa, G.; Castro-Ramirez, L.; Ladera-Castañeda, M.; López-Gurreonero, C.; Cachay-Criado, H.; Aliaga-Mariñas, A.; Cornejo-Pinto, A.; Cervantes-Ganoza, L.; Cayo-Rojas, C.F. The Microhardness and Surface Roughness Assessment of Bulk-Fill Resin Composites Treated with and without the Application of an Oxygen-Inhibited Layer and a Polishing System: An In Vitro Study. *Polymers* **2022**, *14*, 3053. [CrossRef] [PubMed]
16. Szalewski, L.; Wójcik, D.; Bogucki, M.; Szkutnik, J.; Różyło-Kalinowska, I. The Influence of Popular Beverages on Mechanical Properties of Composite Resins. *Materials* **2021**, *14*, 3097. [CrossRef] [PubMed]
17. Gawriołek, M.; Sikorska, E.; Ferreira, L.F.V.; Costa, A.I.; Khmelinskii, I.; Krawczyk, A.; Sikorski, M.; Koczorowski, R. Color and Luminescence Stability of Selected Dental Materials In Vitro: Color and Luminescence Stability. *J. Prosthodont.* **2012**, *21*, 112–122. [CrossRef] [PubMed]
18. Kumari, C.; Bhat, K.; Bansal, R.; Singh, N.; Anupama, A.; Lavanya, T. Evaluation of surface roughness and hardness of newer nanoposterior composite resins after immersion in food-simulating liquids. *Contemp. Clin. Dent.* **2019**, *10*, 289–293. [CrossRef]
19. Hamdy, T.M.; Abdelnabi, A.; Othman, M.S.; Bayoumi, R.E.; Abdelraouf, R.M. Effect of Different Mouthwashes on the Surface Microhardness and Color Stability of Dental Nanohybrid Resin Composite. *Polymers* **2023**, *15*, 815. [CrossRef]
20. Barve, D.; Dave, P.N.; Gulve, M.N.; Sahib, M.A.M.; Naz, F.; Shahabe, S.A. Effect of Commonly Consumed Beverages on Microhardness of Two Types of Composites. *Int. J. Clin. Pediatr. Dent.* **2020**, *13*, 663–667. [CrossRef]
21. Ünal, M.; Candan, M.; İpek, I.; Küçükoflaz, M.; Özer, A. Evaluation of the microhardness of different resin-based dental restorative materials treated with gastric acid: Scanning electron microscopy–energy dispersive X-ray spectroscopy analysis. *Microsc. Res. Tech.* **2021**, *84*, 2140–2148. [CrossRef]

22. Vecek, N.N.; Par, M.; Sever, E.K.; Miletic, I.; Krmek, S.J. The Effect of a Green Smoothie on Microhardness, Profile Roughness andng Color Change of Dental Restorative Materials. *Polymers* **2022**, *14*, 2067. [CrossRef] [PubMed]
23. Fernandes, R.A.; Strazzi-Sahyon, H.B.; Suzuki, T.Y.U.; Briso, A.L.F.; dos Santos, P.H. Effect of dental bleaching on the microhardness and surface roughness of sealed composite resins. *Restor. Dent. Endod.* **2020**, *45*, e12. [CrossRef] [PubMed] [PubMed Central]
24. Camilotti, V.; Detogni, A.C.; Ambrosano, G.M.B.; Mendonça, M.J.; Ueda, J.K.; De Goes, M.F. Effect of acidic solutions present in the diet on the surface roughness of microhybrid composite resins. *Res. Soc. Dev.* **2022**, *11*, e46111426588. [CrossRef]
25. Tavangar, M.; Bagheri, R.; Kwon, T.; Mese, A.; Manton, D.J. Influence of beverages and surface roughness on the color change of resin composites. *J. Investig. Clin. Dent.* **2018**, *9*, e12333. [CrossRef] [PubMed]
26. Patnana, A.K.; Vaidya, N.; Kumar, P.; Pathak, K.; Punia, S.K.; Choudhary, A. Comparative evaluation of the influence of different sports/energy drinks and alcoholic beverages on the surface roughness of three different flowable esthetic restorative materials: An in vitro Analysis. *J. Int. Soc. Prev. Community Dent.* **2020**, *10*, 585–590. [CrossRef]
27. Lepri, C.P.; Palma-Dibb, R.G. Surface roughness and color change of a composite: Influence of beverages and brushing. *Dent. Mater. J.* **2012**, *31*, 689–696. [CrossRef] [PubMed]
28. Sideridou, I.D.; Karabela, M.M.; Vouvoudi, E.C. Physical properties of current dental nanohybrid and nanofill light-cured resin composites. *Dent. Mater.* **2011**, *27*, 598–607. [CrossRef]
29. Szalewski, L.; Szalewska, M.; Jarosz, P.; Woś, M.; Szymańska, J. Temperature Changes in Composite Materials during Photopolymerization. *Appl. Sci.* **2021**, *11*, 474. [CrossRef]
30. Szalewski, L.; Wójcik, D.; Sofińska-Chmiel, W.; Kuśmierz, M.; Różyło-Kalinowska, I. How the Duration and Mode of Photopolymerization Affect the Mechanical Properties of a Dental Composite Resin. *Materials* **2023**, *16*, 113. [CrossRef]

materials

MDPI

Article

How Does Ethylenediaminetetraacetic Acid Irrigation Affect Biodentine? A Multimethod Ex Vivo Study

Katarzyna Dąbrowska [1], Aleksandra Palatyńska-Ulatowska [1,*] and Leszek Klimek [2]

[1] Department of Endodontics, Chair of Conservative Dentistry and Endodontics, Medical University of Lodz, 251 Pomorska Street, 92-217 Lodz, Poland; katarzyna.anna.dabrowska@umed.lodz.pl

[2] Institute of Materials Science and Technology, Technical University of Lodz, 1/15 Stefanowskiego Street, 90-924 Lodz, Poland; leszek.klimek@p.lodz.pl

* Correspondence: aleksandra.palatynska-ulatowska@umed.lodz.pl

Abstract: The activity of biomaterials used during endodontic treatment can be affected by various factors. One of them is the chemical action of the irrigant that they are exposed to. The aim of this multimethod ex vivo study was to evaluate the influence of ethylenediaminetetraacetic acid (EDTA) on the surface appearance and chemical composition of Biodentine used in perforation repair. Twenty material specimens were prepared according to manufacturers' recommendations and divided into two setting-time-based groups, tested after 45 min (group A) and 24 h (group B) of setting. Material was irrigated with 17% EDTA solution with or without simultaneous ultrasonic activation. The surface characteristics and the chemical composition analysis of the Biodentine specimens were performed with the aid of a scanning electron microscope (SEM) and an energy dispersive spectroscopy (EDS) method, respectively. The volumetric loss of material was measured by dedicated digital software in an optical microscope. Statistical analysis was performed. The EDS study confirmed that after the rinsing protocol, the percentage content of elements differed between the groups. The EDTA rinse, whether ultrasonically activated or not, visibly affected the surface appearance and chemical composition of Biodentine. The specimens' surface subjected to irrigation was more irregular under SEM than in a control group. The US activation of the liquid amplified its impact on the tested material. The average volume loss in group A after 5 min irrigation was 3.98 μm^3 for each μm^2 of the chosen area and it increased up to 7.74 $\mu m^3/\mu m^2$ after the ultrasonic activation. In group B, indicated volume loss values were 6.30 and 11.70 $\mu m^3/\mu m^2$ for 5 min irrigation without and with US activation, respectively. Using a 20 min irrigation time and ultrasonic activation increased it up to 32.71 $\mu m^3/\mu m^2$. Each rinsing protocol involving irrigation with ethylenediaminetetraacetic acid modified the surface features and the chemical composition of the evaluated hydraulic tricalcium silicate cement. Further research is needed to indicate the possible impact of the observed changes on its long-term clinical performance.

Keywords: Biodentine; EDTA; energy dispersive spectroscopy; irrigation; perforation; scanning electron microscope; ultrasonic activation

1. Introduction

Complicated endodontic cases, such as chamber floor or furcal perforations, often require the use of highly specified materials, that should efficiently seal the defect and heal the wounded area without harming the contacting intraosseous environment [1]. For the last 25 years a Portland-cement-based mineral trioxide aggregate (MTA) has been used with success for this purpose [2]. The evolution of this material has led to the creation of the whole bioceramic group of dressing cements. Their therapeutic properties, biocompatibility and antimicrobial activity, all deriving from a specific chemical composition, are essential to ensure treatment success [3]. Nevertheless, proper material management is of equal importance. Hence, the clinicians' ability to correctly choose and use these biocements needs to be evaluated and updated.

Biodentine (Septodont, Saint-Maur-des-Fosées, France), also known as "dentine replacement" material [4,5], is a representative of these reparative cements. It is a hydraulic self-setting tricalcium silicate cement with many clinical applications. Biodentine is used in direct and indirect pulp capping [6–8], pulpotomy procedures [9,10], perforation repair [2,11], treatment of immature teeth or an open apex [2,10], root-end retrograde surgical filling [2,12] and as a dentin replacement material [13]. Compared to MTA, it has a shorter setting time [2,14] and comparable healing and sealing properties [15]. Biodentine's main components are di- and tricalcium silicates, which ensure its bioactivity [16]. The manufacturer also uses zirconium oxide as a radiopacifier, calcium chloride as a setting reaction accelerator, calcium carbonate and oxide as fillers, and a hydrosoluble polymer that acts as a water requirement reductor [17].

Standard endodontic procedure, together with mechanical shaping, involves a thorough chemical preparation with the use of 5.25% sodium hypochlorite (NaOCl), 2% chlorhexidine (CHX) and chelating agents—17% ethylenediaminetetraacetic acid (EDTA) or 40% citric acid (CA). This is a crucial part of the canal space disinfection. For the same reason, in more complicated cases of root canal or chamber perforations, constant irrigation following the placement of bioceramic material is required. Endodontic space perforation is a pathogenic or iatrogenic communication between the root canal system and the external tooth surface [18]. The prognosis largely depends on immediate and proper treatment [19]. It often requires the placement of the bioactive material in the first place, e.g., to stop bleeding. The following root canal treatment is performed after closure of the defect. Therefore, the material used for this procedure will be exposed to, among other things, chemical action of the irrigants used after its placement. The cement resistance depends on its setting stage in the moment of irrigation as well as the characteristics of the irrigant. Immediate irrigation may negatively affect the clinical performance of the biocement used for perforation closure [20,21].

This research includes ethylenediaminetetraacetic acid as a rinsing solution used in the final irrigation protocol. It is a chelator able to dissolve inorganic structures by binding calcium and magnesium ions and replacing them with sodium ions [22]. Although its chelating nature is highly required in removing the smear layer and exposing dentinal tubules for better sealer adaptation [23], it may pose a threat to any biocement exposed to it.

There are various irrigation techniques and methods to enhance the standard irrigation procedure. The most common is ultrasonic activation of the rinsing liquid, known as passive ultrasonic irrigation (PUI). The acoustic streaming produced at the tip of the device can remove debris from the canal walls and rupture any aggregations of bacteria [24]. This process is additionally supported by microcavitation and temperature rise in the irrigating solution [25].

The aim of this research was to analyze the influence of ethylenediaminetetraacetic acid used as an irrigant in endodontic procedures, either ultrasonically activated or not, on Biodentine surface appearance and its chemical composition. The volumetric loss of material was evaluated, which is a novelty of this study. Scarce literature on this topic makes the study the first of its kind. The null hypothesis of no differences between different irrigation protocols was adopted.

2. Materials and Methods

Biodentine cement was prepared following the manufacturer's instructions. The powder–liquid ratio, mixing time and method were strictly respected: 5 drops of the dedicated liquid were added vertically to the capsule containing the powder. The capsule was closed and mixed for 30 s in a mixing device (Dental Mixer SYG200, Septodont, Saint-Maur-des-Fosées, France) at a speed of 4000 rpm. Mixed material was placed in polyvinyl tubes (polyvinyl chloride—PVC; Cellfast, Stalowa Wola, Poland) and compacted with the aid of a plugger on a smooth glass plate. The specimens were divided into two setting-time-based groups: group A—investigated after 45 min, group B—after 24 h of setting. After designated times, the material was cautiously removed from the forms. Biodentine specimens were then dry-polished with rotating sandpapers with subsequent grits from 600 to 1200 in order to equalize the investigated surfaces. Twenty standardized cylindrical specimens of 3 mm height and 8 mm diameter (Figure 1) were prepared this way.

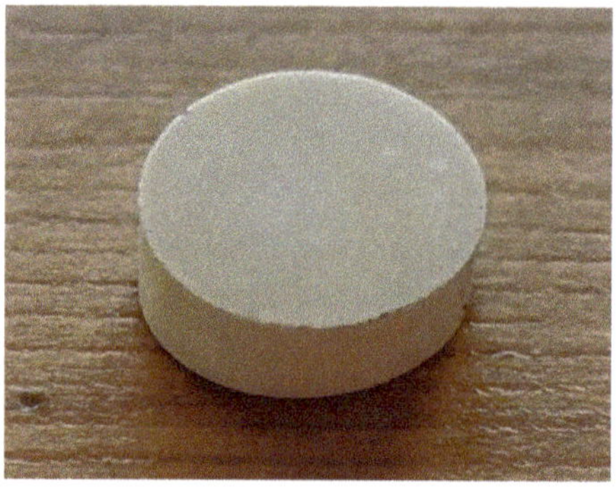

Figure 1. Cylindrical Biodentine specimen.

The specimens were categorized randomly into groups, as shown in Figure 2.

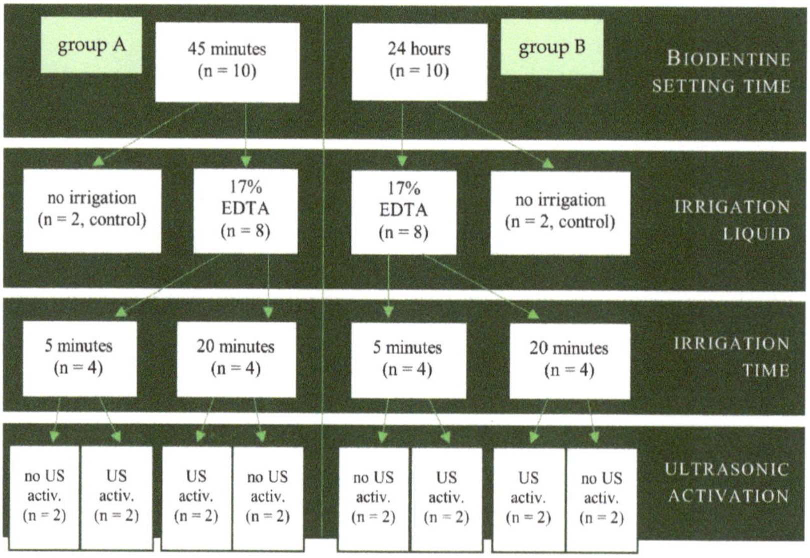

Figure 2. Biodentine specimens' distribution.

The control group consisted of 4 specimens and was not subjected to any irrigation protocol. The research group was rinsed with 10 mL of 17% EDTA (Cerkamed, Stalowa Wola, Poland) for 5 or 20 min, with or without continuous ultrasonic activation in a Sonic-0.5 device (Polsonic, Warsaw, Poland). After each protocol, Biodentine specimens were immersed in demineralized water and lightly dried with compressed air in order to avoid EDTA remnants or any other precipitates on the investigated surfaces.

The surface appearance of each Biodentine specimen, after having been subjected to its designated irrigation protocol, was analyzed in the scanning electron microscope

(SEM, S-3000N, HITACHI, Tokyo, Japan) with a magnification of 1.0 k, 15 kV accelerating voltage and 15 mm working distance on an area of 2 × 3 mm. The chemical composition of the material's surface was examined in SEM using X-ray microanalysis with the energy dispersive spectroscopy method (EDS) with the aid of the Vantage software (Version 4.1, Thermo Fisher Scientific, Waltham, MA, USA) and AZtec software (Version 1.0A, Oxford Instruments, Tubney Woods, Abingdon, UK). The electron beam was automatically set so that the detector could keep up with counting the X-ray quanta. The detector dead time was set at 25–30%. Biodentine volumetric loss was evaluated in an optic microscope VHX-950F with its dedicated digital software (Keyence, Mechelen, Belgium) using 0.5 k magnification. The measurements were taken in 5 randomly chosen areas of each specimen and their arithmetic mean and standard deviation were calculated. Statistical analysis of the obtained results was carried out in order to compare the dependence of the performed rinsing protocol on the loss of material volume. As the specimens did not meet the normality assumption, the Kruskal–Wallis test was used in Statistica 13 software (StatSoft, Tulsa, OK, USA). A p value below 0.05 was deemed significant. The null hypothesis of no differences between different irrigation protocols was adopted.

3. Results

3.1. Biodentine Surface Chemical Composition

The chemical percentage composition of each Biodentine specimen's surface was registered on the basis of the data obtained with the EDS method (Table 1, Figure 3) and spectrograms were created (Figure 4). The results were compared between the groups and with the control group.

The EDS study results indicate the presence of elements specific to Biodentine—peaks of calcium, silicon, carbon, zirconium, chlorine and oxygen are clearly visible on the spectrograms.

The results show that the irrigation protocol with EDTA changes the chemical composition of the tested material and differences between the control and the investigated groups occur. Changes are also detectable when comparing the specimens after two setting times (group A and B) and the specimens subjected to ultrasonic irrigation.

Table 1. Atom percentage [%] of Biodentine specimens' surface in control group, group A (after 45 min setting time) and in group B (after 24 h setting time).

Element	45 min Setting Time					24 h Setting Time				
	No Irrigation	17% EDTA 5 min	17% EDTA 20 min	17% EDTA + US 5 min	17% EDTA + US 20 min	No Irrigation	17% EDTA 5 min	17% EDTA 20 min	17% EDTA + US 5 min	17% EDTA + US 20 min
Carbon	11.35	15.0	21.1	17.5	18.8	10.41	18.0	15.5	15.8	14.9
Oxygen	49.61	44.1	44.2	48.1	46.3	49.93	41.9	44.7	44.6	44.0
Silicon	5.96	7.0	12.5	11.1	17.2	9.09	3.1	3.6	3.4	7.5
Zirconium	0.56	2.5	3.2	3.4	3.8	0.74	1.,5	9.7	6.4	7.7
Chlorine	3.64	0.3	0.6	0.9	0.3	2.09	0.5	0.3	0.2	0.5
Calcium	28.87	29.9	17.5	18.7	12.9	27.74	23.4	24.2	28.0	15.2
Natrium	0.0	1.2	0.9	0.3	0.6	0.0	0.8	1.1	1.2	8.8
Iron	0.0	0.0	0.0	0.0	0.0	0.0	0.3	0.3	0.2	0.3
Aluminum	0.0	0.0	0.0	0.0	0.1	0.0	0.0	0.0	0.0	0.1
Magnesium	0.0	0.0	0.0	0.0	0.0	0.0	0.4	0.6	0.3	1.1

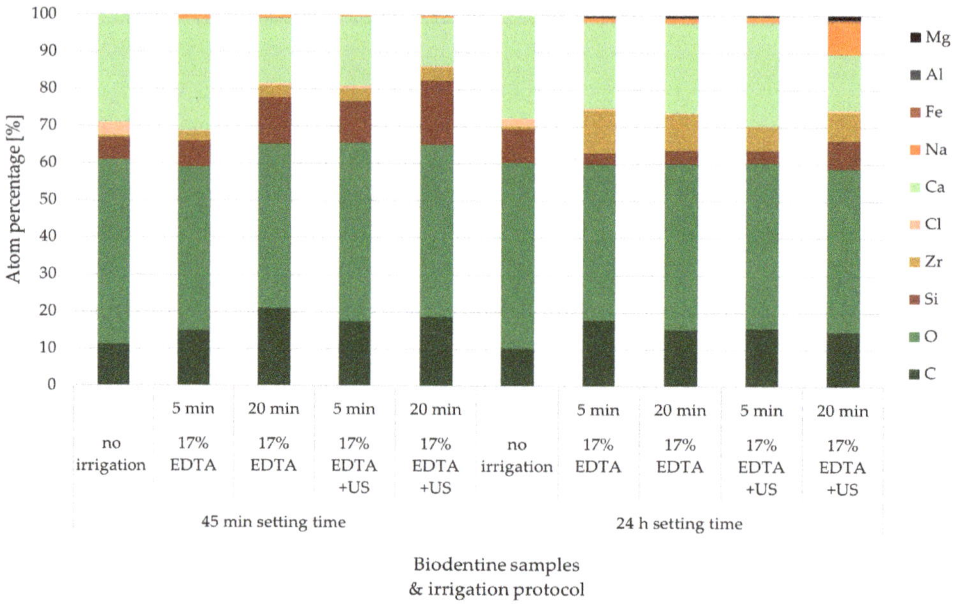

Figure 3. Changes in the chemical composition of Biodentine specimens' surface after different irrigation protocols involving 17% sodium edetate solution.

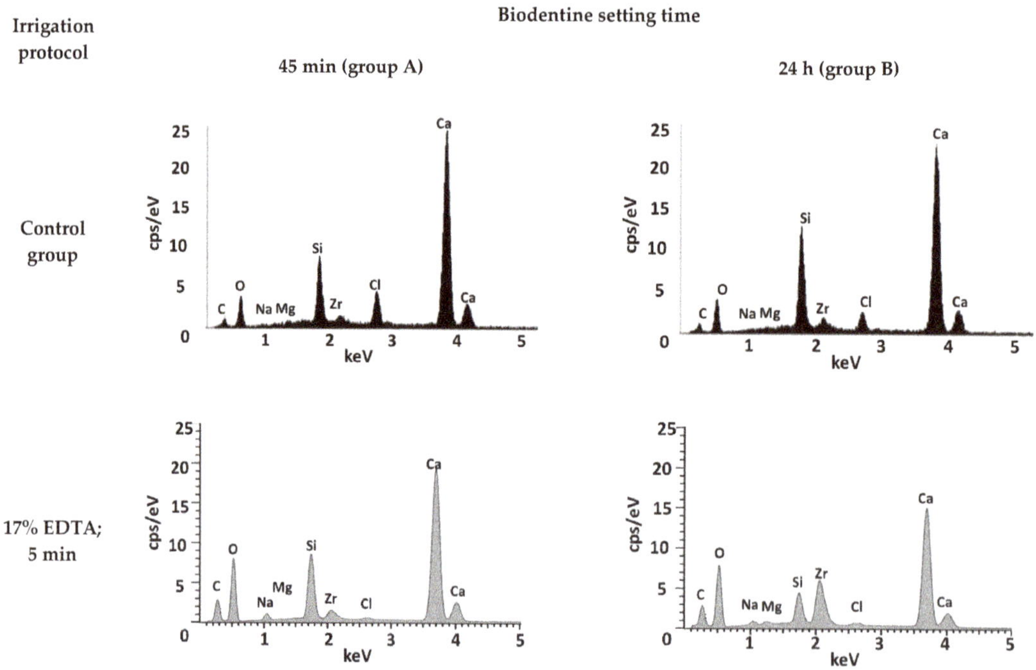

Figure 4. *Cont.*

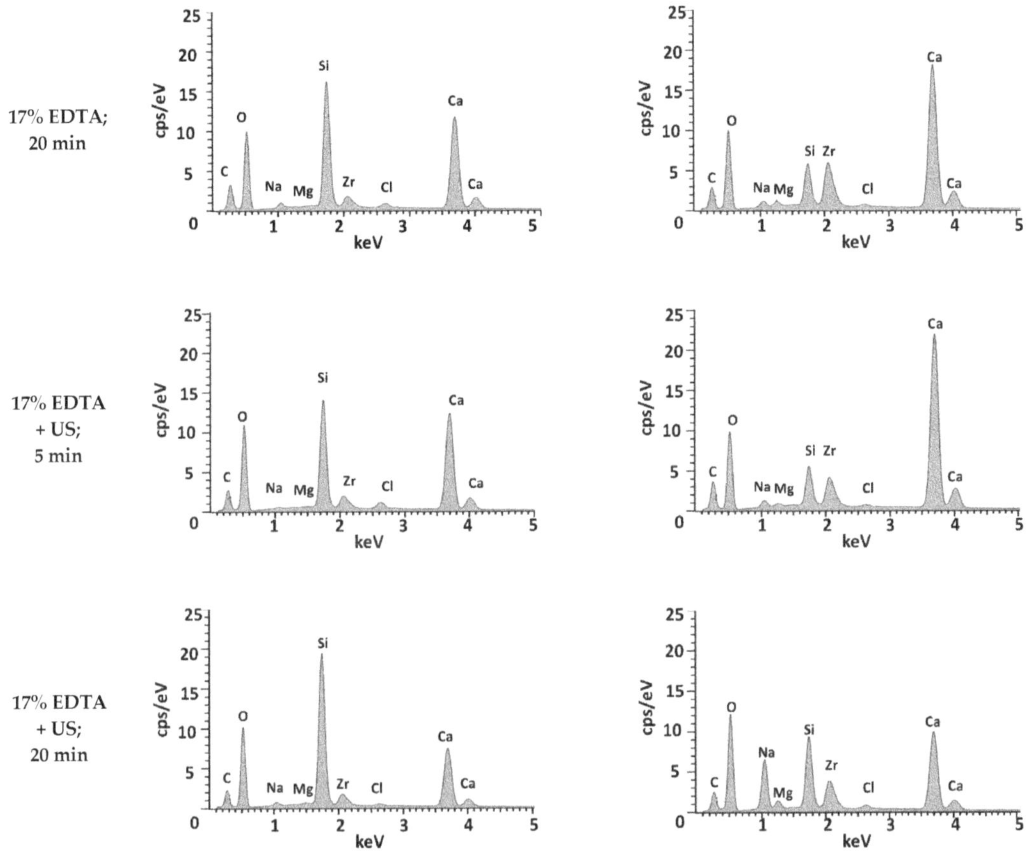

Figure 4. EDS spectrograms of Biodentine specimens.

Within specimens from group A, a trend was observed in the percentage of calcium. Its content decreased with the elongation of the rinsing time and after ultrasonic activation in favor of an increase in the percentage of silicon. The most pronounced change in the proportion of calcium was visible in the specimens from group B subjected to the longest rinsing protocol with US activation. In specimens from both setting time groups, an increasing percentage of zirconium was noted, with a clearer tendency in the specimens after the longer setting time (group B). It can therefore be concluded that both the longer time of irrigation and the use of ultrasonic activation enhance the chelating effect of ethylenediaminetetraacetic acid. The longer the setting time of Biodentine cement, the better its resistance to this action.

In comparison with the control group, the effect of irrigation protocols using 17% sodium edetate can be seen in almost every specimen. Only the specimens evaluated after the shortest setting and rinsing time without ultrasonic activation are similar in composition to the control. In the group A, the tendencies of changes are clear—the prolonged rinsing time with ethylenediaminetetraacetic acid as well as the use of ultrasonic activation decrease the percentage of calcium and chlorine, in opposition to zirconium and silicon in the surface composition of Biodentine. In specimens from group B, a decrease in the content of chlorine and silicon and an increase in zirconium percentage is detectable. A simultaneous decrease in the calcium level was only noticed in Biodentine specimens after the longest setting and rinsing time with ultrasonic activation.

3.2. Biodentine Surface Appearance

SEM images of Biodentine specimens from both setting time groups were compared. The obtained results indicate the influence of 17% EDTA solution on the surface appearance of the investigated material when compared with the control specimens (Figure 5).

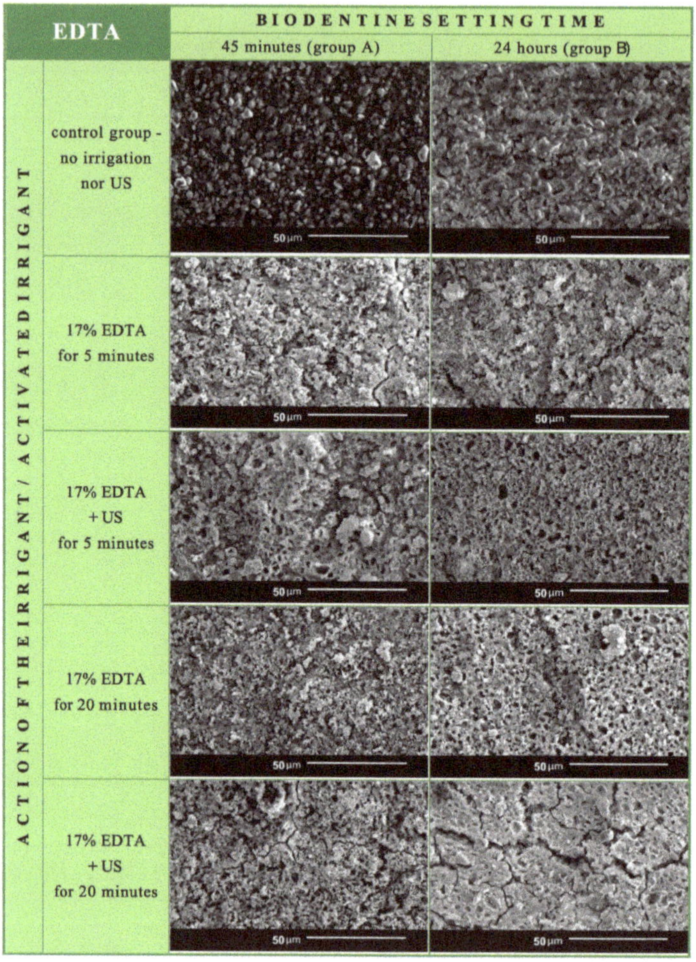

Figure 5. Biodentine specimens' surface visualized in SEM.

The effect of the irrigation protocol with 17% EDTA solution was visible on each tested specimen. The Biodentine surface was more irregular than in the control group. The material with hollow pits and round-shaped defects resembled the etched dentin with open tubules.

Specimens with longer irrigation exposure time were more affected than those after 5 min of rinsing. The ultrasonic activation also enhanced the chelating action of the tested irrigant. Although this result was noticeable in both setting time groups, Biodentine after 24 h setting seemed more susceptible to liquid action.

In both groups A and B, the longest irrigation time with ultrasonic activation resulted in the most pronounced changes on the surface of the cement. It became very irregular, with crystals "torn" from its surface.

3.3. Biodentine Surface Volume Loss

The specimens' surface visualized as 2D color maps are shown in Figure 6.

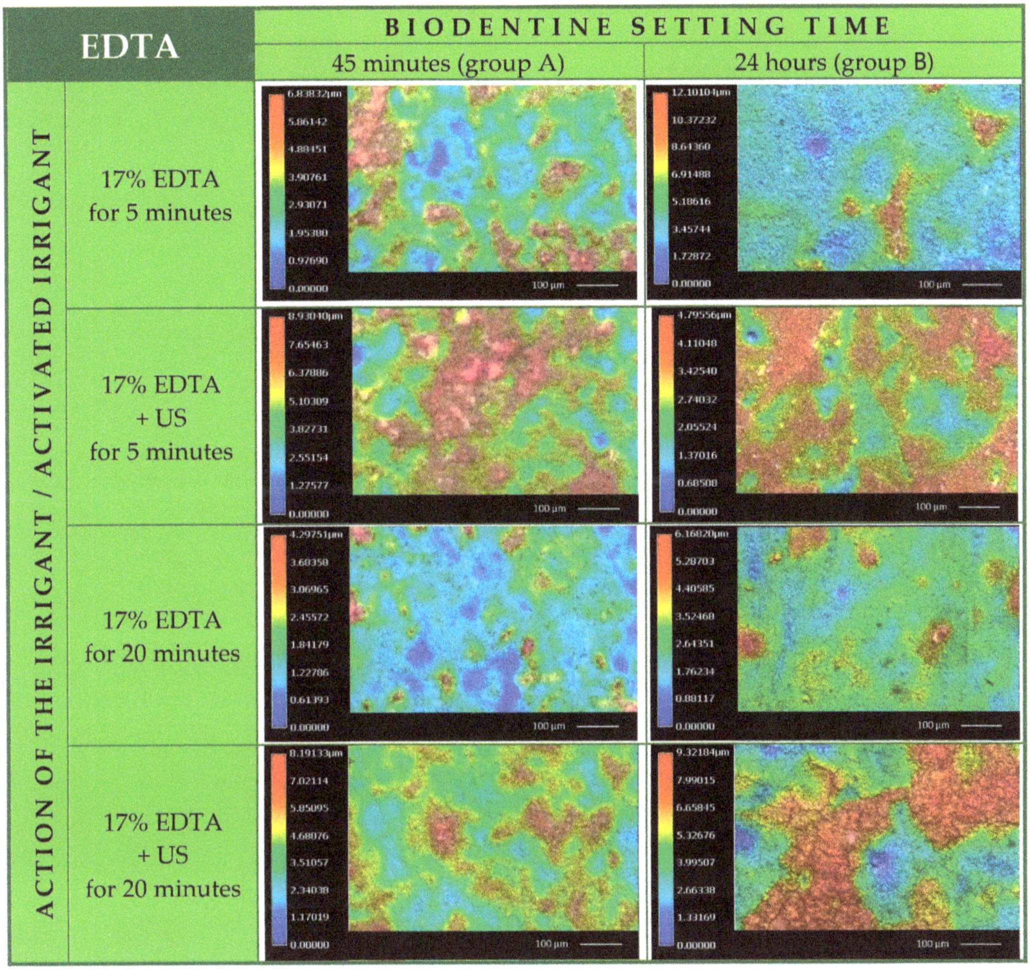

Figure 6. 2D color map of Biodentine surface of the specimens from group A and B after irrigation with 17% EDTA with and without ultrasonic activation.

The mean values of total volume loss, volume loss per 1 μm^2 and standard deviation of each Biodentine specimen are presented in Table 2.

In the specimens from group A, the average volume loss after 5 min irrigation with EDTA was 3.98 μm^3 for each μm^2 of surface. After 5 min of rinsing with ethylenediaminetetraacetic acid with ultrasonic activation, the loss was higher: 7.74 μm^3/μm^2. For specimens subjected to a 20 min EDTA irrigation, the loss was 2.95 μm^3 per μm^2, whereas ultrasonic activation increased this value to 6.57 μm^3/μm^2.

In the specimens from group B, the loss of volume was increasing with the increase in rinsing intensity. After 5 min of EDTA irrigation, the volume loss was 6.30 μm^3 for each μm^2 of surface area. After 5 min with ultrasonic activation, the loss was higher: 11.70 μm^3/μm^2. For specimens subjected to 20 min irrigation with sodium edetate, the volume loss was 10.64 μm^3 per μm^2, and ultrasonic activation increased this value to 32.71 μm^3/μm^2.

Table 2. The mean values of total volume loss, volume loss per 1 μm^2 and standard deviation [μm^3] in Biodentine specimens after EDTA irrigation with or without US activation.

Parameter	Irrigation Protocol				
	No Irrigation (Control)	**17% EDTA 5 min**	**17% EDTA 20 min**	**17% EDTA + US 5 min**	**17% EDTA + US 20 min**
	Group A—45 min Setting				
total volume loss	602,927.89 μm^3	417,313.69 μm^3	295,658.41 μm^3	811,488.96 μm^3	692,396.96 μm^3
volume loss per 1 μm^2	5.03 μm^3	3.98 μm^3	2.95 μm^3	7.74 μm^3	6.57 μm^3
standard deviation	298,351.33 μm^3	99,037.94 μm^3	54,593.00 μm^3	242,789.08 μm^3	166,958.76 μm^3
	Group B—24 h Setting				
total volume loss	602,927.89 μm^3	660,091.36 μm^3	1,012,729.76 μm^3	1,115,836.11 μm^3	3,394,783.66 μm^3
volume loss per 1 μm^2	5.03 μm^3	6.30 μm^3	10.64 μm^3	11.70 μm^3	32.71 μm^3
standard deviation	298,351.33 μm^3	196,107.81 μm^3	302,416.00 μm^3	256,712.78 μm^3	738,214.44 μm^3

Comparing the results to the baseline situation (control group without any irrigation), there was practically no effect of EDTA irrigation on the specimens from group A or on the specimen from group B rinsed for 5 min without US activation.

The statistical analysis of the obtained results is presented in Table 3 and in Figure 7 and shows the dependance of material volume loss from the chosen irrigation protocol. The Kruskal–Wallis test was used, where the volume loss [μm^3] was the dependent variable and the irrigation protocol—the independent variable. Statistically significant differences were marked ($p < 0.05000$).

The results of the Kruskal–Wallis test ($p = 0.0001$), at the assumed level of significance ($\alpha = 0.05$), indicate the rejection of the null hypothesis.

Table 3. Statistical analysis—comparison of the effect of different irrigation protocols with 17% EDTA on the volume loss of Biodentine. Statistically significant differences ($p < 0.0500$) marked in italics.

		Group A				Group B			
		17% EDTA, 5 min	**17% EDTA, 20 min**	**17% EDTA + US, 5 min**	**17% EDTA + US, 20 min**	**17% EDTA, 5 min**	**17% EDTA, 20 min**	**17% EDTA + US, 5 min**	**17% EDTA + US, 20 min**
group A	17% EDTA, 5 min		1.0000	1.0000	1.0000	1.0000	0.3591	0.1064	*0.0014*
	17% EDTA, 20 min	1.0000		0.5023	1.0000	1.0000	0.0750	*0.0183*	*0.0001*
	17% EDTA + US, 5 min	1.0000	0.5023		1.0000	1.0000	1.0000	1.0000	0.7695
	17% EDTA + US, 20 min	1.0000	1.0000	1.0000		1.0000	1.0000	1.0000	0.2533
group B	17% EDTA, 5 min	1.0000	1.0000	1.0000	1.0000		1.0000	1.0000	0.1623
	17% EDTA, 20 min	0.3591	0.0750	1.0000	1.0000	1.0000		1.0000	1.0000
	17% EDTA + US, 5 min	0.1064	*0.0183*	1.0000	1.0000	1.0000	1.0000		1.0000
	17% EDTA + US, 20 min	*0.0014*	*0.0001*	0.7695	0.2533	0.1623	1.0000	1.0000	

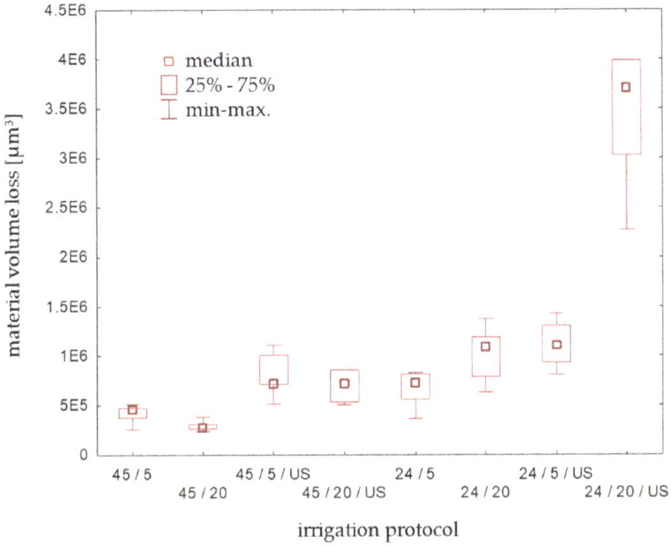

Figure 7. Statistical analysis—graphical comparison of the effect of different irrigation protocols using 17% EDTA on the volume loss of Biodentine. (45/5 = 45 min setting time, 5 min irrigation; 24/20/US = 24 h setting time, 20 min irrigation with ultrasonic activation etc.).

Statistically significant differences were found between borderline specimens: 45 min setting time, 5 min vs. 24 h setting time, 20 min irrigation with 17% EDTA ultrasonically activated as well as the Biodentine specimen from group A, after 20 min EDTA irrigation vs. specimens from group B after 20 min and 5 min EDTA irrigation with US activation. No clear trend was detected for any tested irrigation protocol.

4. Discussion

Biocompatibility and sealing properties of the modern biocements used in endodontics are the crucial features corresponding to the quality of the treatment and its success rate. Nevertheless, the material management is equally significant. It is essential for a clinician to know about the indications, adequate management and application techniques of biomaterials to ensure long-term treatment success. This research is therefore clinically relevant.

A perforation repair material should have adequately high dislodgement resistance to withstand the functional forces and forces of condensation [26]. The contact of perforation repair material with various irrigants and blood can inadvertently modify their physical properties and consequently affect the treatment outcome. According to Sethi et al., Biodentine showed maximum cohesive failures (62.5%) followed by mixed (20.8%) and adhesive failures (16.7%) [27]. The presented analysis of the cement features seems to confirm that observation. In the literature, the shear bond strength and push-out bond strength tests are the most often proposed to assess the dislodgement resistance of perforation repair materials in endodontics. The connection quality between Biodentine and dentin and its compressive strength or color stability are widely evaluated [28,29]. However, the impact of canal rinsing agents and their ultrasonic activation on Biodentine surface is less likely described. In some studies, the EDTA was not even included in the tested irrigation protocols [30]. Measurement of the volume loss of the material after the irrigation protocol with this chelator is the novelty of this trial.

Biodentine specimens were segregated on the basis of selected setting times [17]. The setting time recommended by the manufacturer—12 min [31]—was verified as too short for the analysis. The material was not set enough to withstand the protocol of irrigation and became completely disintegrated during the irrigation. That fact has made it impossible to continue the experiment in this group of specimens. Although it is supposed to be sufficient in conservative dentistry procedures [32,33], the degradation of the material surface may have a negative effect on the endodontic therapy outcome. After 12 min of setting, the cement was not yet able to withstand the immediate irrigation protocol, especially with US activation.

Rinsing with chelators is essential for the removal of the smear layer in the final part of chemo-mechanical cleaning and shaping of the canal space. From the clinical point of view, chelating irrigation liquids should be in contact with the dentin for no longer than 3 min in order to reduce canal wall erosion [34,35]. Nevertheless, in calcified, thin and curved canals, EDTA in the form of liquid, cream, gel, paste, etc. is used to obtain the patent canal and to enhance its mechanical cleaning and shaping [36]. Thus, the contact time of the chelator with the dentin and the bioceramic material placed in the endodontic space may be much longer. Therefore, the choice of prolonged irrigation times for this trial is still justified. Moreover, the presented results are part of the bigger project, comparing the data of the action of other agents, e.g., sodium hypochlorite. It was also the reason for choosing longer times of irrigation protocols (5 and 20 min). Group A consisted of Biodentine specimens set in a 45 min irrigation time, as indicated by Grech et al. [37]. After EDTA irrigation, the surface was visually affected. The material did not seem to be fully set, which can be explained by the standard behavior of cement and its setting mechanism. In accordance with the American Society for Testing and Materials (ASTM) standards, it is divided into two stages: initial setting and maturation or final setting. The initial phase lasts until the material starts losing its plasticity. The final phase ends when the cement becomes rigid, which means that with the application of increasing stress, it fractures rather than flows [38]. Biodentine derives from Portland cement, so its setting behavior resembles much the above described.

The material in group B was setting for a longer time, yet still the irrigation with 17% EDTA solution caused partial disintegration of the material surface. The ultrasonic activation as well as the increase in irrigation time seemed to amplify the EDTA effect on Biodentine more visibly than in specimens from group A. Taking the presented results and all of the above into consideration, it can therefore be concluded that both the longer time of irrigation and the use of ultrasonic activation enhance the chelating effect of ethylenediaminetetraacetic acid. The longer the setting time of Biodentine cement, the better its resistance to this action.

Numerous cracks could be noticed on the material surface visualized in SEM. Most probably, they were created as a result of the testing procedure, which involved obtaining a vacuum in the SEM chamber. This did not affect the volume microscopy measurements, as the tested spots on the Biodentine surface were consciously chosen by the operator.

The interpretation of EDS analysis needs to be carried out bearing in mind that the software equalizes the results up to 100%. This means that the increased percentage of a certain component leads to the decreased percentage of another, but not necessarily the actual decrease in number or volume. Taking into account the chelating nature of the tested irrigant, the loss of calcium is obvious. EDTA incorporates the mineral ion into a hydrosoluble complex or chelate [39]. The consequential rise in silicon level arises from the chemical breakdown of the tricalcium silicates formed by both elements. After irrigating the set material with EDTA, with the partial removal of calcium from the system comes the need to equalize the overall percentage to 100% by the software; hence, the increase in the calculated amount of silicon.

The obtained modifications in the percentage of elements in the surface composition of the tested specimens are only a preliminary indicator of the changes that occur in the material. The volume loss analysis included various measurement points on the specimens, which makes the statistics valid; nevertheless, obtaining data from a greater number of specimens is still a direction for further research.

This study is limited by its ex vivo form. An observation and analysis of the clinical behavior of Biodentine in endodontic procedures following perforation closure is highly advisable as a direction of future research.

5. Conclusions

Irrigation with EDTA solution, either ultrasonically activated or not, visibly affected the surface appearance of Biodentine. The chemical composition of the tested material was also altered. The effect is more visible after US activation of the irrigant. That is why the continuation of endodontic procedures involving irrigation with EDTA straight after Biodentine placement is not recommended. Further research is needed to evaluate the potential of the material changes described in this paper to alter the clinical outcome of the treatment.

Author Contributions: Conceptualization, K.D. and A.P.-U.; methodology, L.K.; software, K.D. and L.K.; validation, K.D., A.P.-U. and L.K.; investigation, K.D. and L.K.; resources, K.D., L.K. and A.P.-U.; data curation, K.D.; writing—original draft preparation, K.D.; writing—review and editing, K.D., L.K. and A.P.-U.; visualization, K.D.; supervision, A.P.-U. and L.K.; project administration, K.D. and A.P.-U.; funding acquisition, K.D. and A.P.-U. All authors have read and agreed to the published version of the manuscript.

Funding: This work was supported by a grant No 503/2-044-02/503-21-001-18 from Medical University of Lodz. It was carried out as part of doctoral research supported by the project: "InterChemMed—Interdisciplinary Doctoral Studies of Łódź Public Universities", co-financed by the European Social Fund under Measure 3.2. Doctoral Studies of Priority Axis III Higher Education for the Economy and Development of the Operational Programme Knowledge Education Development 2014-2020 (POWR.03.02.00-00-I029/16).

Institutional Review Board Statement: Not applicable.

Informed Consent Statement: Not applicable.

Data Availability Statement: Data are contained within the article.

Conflicts of Interest: The authors declare that there are no conflicts of interest regarding the publication of this paper.

References

1. Dawood, A.E.; Parashos, P.; Wong, R.H.K.; Reynolds, E.C.; Manton, D.J. Calcium Silicate-Based Cements: Composition, Properties, and Clinical Applications. *J. Investig. Clin. Dent.* **2017**, *8*, e12195. [CrossRef]
2. Torabinejad, M.; Parirokh, M.; Dummer, P.M.H. Mineral Trioxide Aggregate and Other Bioactive Endodontic Cements: An Updated Overview—Part II: Other Clinical Applications and Complications. *Int. Endod. J.* **2018**, *51*, 284–317. [CrossRef]
3. Falkowska, J.; Chady, T.; Dura, W.; Droździk, A.; Tomasik, M.; Marek, E.; Safranow, K.; Lipski, M. The Washout Resistance of Bioactive Root-End Filling Materials. *Materials* **2023**, *16*, 5757. [CrossRef]
4. Jitaru, S.; Hodisan, I.; Timis, L.; Lucian, A.; Bud, M. The Use of Bioceramics in Endodontics—Literature Review. *Clujul Med.* **2016**, *89*, 470–473. [CrossRef]
5. Khan, A.S.; Syed, M.R. A Review of Bioceramics-Based Dental Restorative Materials. *Dent. Mater. J.* **2019**, *38*, 163–176. [CrossRef]
6. Camilleri, J. Hydration Characteristics of Biodentine and Theracal Used as Pulp Capping Materials. *Dent. Mater.* **2014**, *30*, 709–715. [CrossRef] [PubMed]
7. Awawdeh, L.; Al-Qudah, A.; Hamouri, H.; Chakra, R.J. Outcomes of Vital Pulp Therapy Using Mineral Trioxide Aggregate or Biodentine: A Prospective Randomized Clinical Trial. *J. Endod.* **2018**, *44*, 1603–1609. [CrossRef] [PubMed]
8. Kunert, M.; Lukomska-Szymanska, M. Bio-Inductive Materials in Direct and Indirect Pulp Capping—A Review Article. *Materials* **2020**, *13*, 1204. [CrossRef] [PubMed]
9. Cuadros-Fernández, C.; Lorente Rodríguez, A.I.; Sáez-Martínez, S.; García-Binimelis, J.; About, I.; Mercadé, M. Short-Term Treatment Outcome of Pulpotomies in Primary Molars Using Mineral Trioxide Aggregate and Biodentine: A Randomized Clinical Trial. *Clin. Oral Investig.* **2016**, *20*, 1639–1645. [CrossRef] [PubMed]
10. Taha, N.A.; Abdulkhader, S.Z. Full Pulpotomy with Biodentine in Symptomatic Young Permanent Teeth with Carious Exposure. *J. Endod.* **2018**, *44*, 932–937. [CrossRef] [PubMed]
11. About, I. Biodentine: From Biochemical and Bioactive Properties to Clinical Applications. *G. Ital. Endod.* **2016**, *30*, 81–88. [CrossRef]

12. Caron, G.; Azérad, J.; Faure, M.O.; Machtou, P.; Boucher, Y. Use of a New Retrograde Filling Material (Biodentine) for Endodontic Surgery: Two Case Reports. *Int. J. Oral Sci.* **2014**, *6*, 250–253. [CrossRef]
13. Camilleri, J. Investigation of Biodentine as Dentine Replacement Material. *J. Dent.* **2013**, *41*, 600–610. [CrossRef]
14. Parirokh, M.; Torabinejad, M.; Dummer, P.M.H. Mineral Trioxide Aggregate and Other Bioactive Endodontic Cements: An Updated Overview—Part I: Vital Pulp Therapy. *Int. Endod. J.* **2018**, *51*, 177–205. [CrossRef]
15. Solanki, N.; Venkappa, K.; Shah, N. Biocompatibility and Sealing Ability of Mineral Trioxide Aggregate and Biodentine as Root-End Filling Material: A Systematic Review. *J. Conserv. Dent.* **2018**, *21*, 10–15. [PubMed]
16. Camilleri, J.; Grech, L.; Galea, K.; Keir, D.; Fenech, M.; Formosa, L.; Damidot, D.; Mallia, B. Porosity and Root Dentine to Material Interface Assessment of Calcium Silicate-Based Root-End Filling Materials. *Clin. Oral Investig.* **2014**, *18*, 1437–1446. [CrossRef]
17. Buła, K.; Palatyńska-Ulatowska, A.; Klimek, L. Biodentine Management and Setting Time with Vicat and Vickers Evaluation; a Survey-Based Study on Clinicians' Experience. *Arch. Mater. Sci. Eng.* **2020**, *103*, 75–85. [CrossRef]
18. American Association of Endodontists. AAE Glossary of Endodontic Terms. Available online: https://www.aae.org/specialty/clinical-resources/glossary-endodontic-terms/%0Ahttp://www.nxtbook.com/nxtbooks/aae/endodonticglossary2016/#/0 (accessed on 20 May 2023).
19. Estrela, C.; Decurcio, D. de A.; Rossi-Fedele, G.; Silva, J.A.; Guedes, O.A.; Borges, Á.H. Root Perforations: A Review of Diagnosis, Prognosis and Materials. *Braz. Oral Res.* **2018**, *32*, 133–146. [CrossRef] [PubMed]
20. Palatyńska-Ulatowska, A.; Buła, K.; Klimek, L. Influence of Sodium Hypochlorite and Ultrasounds on Surface Features and Chemical Composition of Biodentine Tricalcium Silicate-Based Material. *Dent. Mater. J.* **2020**, *39*, 587–592. [CrossRef]
21. Dąbrowska, K.; Palatyńska-Ulatowska, A.; Klimek, L. The Effect of Irrigation with Citric Acid on Biodentine Tricalcium Silicate-Based Cement: SEM-EDS In Vitro Study. *Materials* **2022**, *15*, 3467. [CrossRef] [PubMed]
22. Zehnder, M. Root Canal Irrigants. *J. Endod.* **2006**, *32*, 389–398. [CrossRef]
23. de Arruda, J.A.A.; Schuch, L.F.; Pereira, A.; Monteiro, J.L.G.C.; Melo-Júnior, P.M.R.; Mesquita, R.A.; Moreno, A.; Callou, G. Investigation of Different Sodium Hypochlorite Volumes, Concentrations and Times of Irrigation in Endodontic Therapy: A Systematic Review. *Arch. Health Investig.* **2019**, *8*, 185–191. [CrossRef]
24. Moreira, R.N.; Pinto, E.B.; Galo, R.; Falci, S.G.M.; Mesquita, A.T. Passive Ultrasonic Irrigation in Root Canal: Systematic Review and Meta-Analysis. *Acta Odontol. Scand.* **2019**, *77*, 55–60. [CrossRef]
25. Dioguardi, M.; Di Gioia, G.; Illuzzi, G.; Laneve, E.; Cocco, A.; Troiano, G. Endodontic Irrigants: Different Methods to Improve Efficacy and Related Problems. *Eur. J. Dent.* **2018**, *12*, 459–466. [CrossRef]
26. Ballal, V.; Marques, J.N.; Campos, C.N.; Lima, C.O.; Simão, R.A.; Prado, M. Effects of Chelating Agent and Acids on Biodentine. *Aust. Dent. J.* **2018**, *63*, 170–176. [CrossRef]
27. Sethi, S.; Bhushan, J.; Joshi, R.; Singla, R.; Sidhu, K. Effect of Different Irrigants on the Push-out Bond Strength of Biodentine and TheraCal LC when Used for Perforation Repair in Simulated Condition. *J. Conserv. Dent.* **2023**, *26*, 321–325. [CrossRef] [PubMed]
28. Rebolloso de Barrio, E.; Gancedo-Caravia, L.; García-Barbero, E.; Pérez-Higueras, J.J. Effect of Exposure to Root Canal Irrigants on the Push-out Bond Strength of Calcium Silicate–Based Cements. *Clin. Oral Investig.* **2021**, *25*, 3267–3274. [CrossRef] [PubMed]
29. Elsayed, M.A.; Islam, M.S.; Elbeltagy, K.; Nassar, M. Effect of Different Chelating Agents on the Shear Bond Strength of Calcium Silicate-Based Cements to Coronal Dentin. *Aust. Endod. J.* **2023**, *49*, 426–462. [CrossRef] [PubMed]
30. Eren, S.K.; Örs, S.A.; Aksel, H.; Canay, Ş.; Karasan, D. Effect of Irrigants on the Color Stability, Solubility, and Surface Characteristics of Calcium-Silicate Based Cements. *Restor. Dent. Endod.* **2022**, *47*, e10. [CrossRef] [PubMed]
31. Septodont Biodentine Active Biosilicate Technology Scientific File. In Vitro. 2010. Available online: http://www.oraverse.com/bio/img/Biodentine-ScientificFile.pdf (accessed on 15 May 2020).
32. Borkar, S.A.; Ataide, I. Biodentine Pulpotomy Several Days after Pulp Exposure: Four Case Reports. *J. Conserv. Dent.* **2015**, *18*, 73–78. [CrossRef]
33. Villat, C.; Grosgogeat, B.; Seux, D.; Farge, P. Conservative Approach of a Symptomatic Carious Immature Permanent Tooth Using a Tricalcium Silicate Cement (Biodentine): A Case Report. *Restor. Dent. Endod.* **2013**, *38*, 258–264. [CrossRef]
34. Mai, S.; Kim, Y.K.; Arola, D.D.; Gu, L.S.; Kim, J.R.; Pashley, D.H.; Tay, F.R. Differential Aggressiveness of Ethylenediamine Tetraacetic Acid in Causing Canal Wall Erosion in the Presence of Sodium Hypochlorite. *J. Dent.* **2010**, *38*, 201–206. [CrossRef]
35. Qian, W.; Shen, Y.; Haapasalo, M. Quantitative Analysis of the Effect of Irrigant Solution Sequences on Dentin Erosion. *J. Endod.* **2011**, *37*, 1437–1441. [CrossRef]
36. Chandler, N.; Chellappa, D. Lubrication during Root Canal Treatment. *Aust. Endod. J.* **2019**, *45*, 106–110. [CrossRef] [PubMed]
37. Grech, L.; Mallia, B.; Camilleri, J. Investigation of the Physical Properties of Tricalcium Silicate Cement-Based Root-End Filling Materials. *Dent. Mater.* **2013**, *29*, e20–e28. [CrossRef] [PubMed]
38. *ASTM C125-20*; Standard Terminology Relating to Concrete and Concrete Aggregates. ASTM International: West Conshohocken, PA, USA, 2020; pp. 1–9. [CrossRef]
39. Sears, M.E. Chelation: Harnessing and Enhancing Heavy Metal Detoxification—A Review. *Sci. World J.* **2013**, *2013*, 219840. [CrossRef] [PubMed]

materials

MDPI

Article

Zirconium Oxide as a Novel Material for Post-Endodontically Treated Teeth: Comparative Fracture Behavior of 3D-Printed Cobalt–Chromium, Milled Zirconium Oxide, and Quartz Fiber Posts

Armin Sokolowski [1], Fernando Gustavo Warchomicka [2], Lukas Seebacher [1], Bernhard Remschmidt [3], Marcus Rieder [3], Lumnije Kqiku-Biblekaj [1] and Alwin Sokolowski [1,*]

[1] Division of Restorative Dentistry, Periodontology and Prosthodontics, Department of Dental Medicine and Oral Health, Medical University of Graz, 8010 Graz, Austria; armin.sokolowski@medunigraz.at (A.S.); lukas.seebacher@medunigraz.at (L.S.); lumnije.kqiku@medunigraz.at (L.K.-B.)

[2] Institute of Materials Science, Joining and Forming, Graz University of Technology, 8010 Graz, Austria; fernando.warchomicka@tugraz.at

[3] Division of Oral and Maxillofacial Surgery, Department of Dental Medicine and Oral Health, Medical University of Graz, 8010 Graz, Austria; bernhard.remschmidt@medunigraz.at (B.R.); marcus.rieder@medunigraz.at (M.R.)

* Correspondence: alwin.sokolowski@medunigraz.at; Tel.: +43-316-385-30678

Abstract: This study evaluates the mechanical properties of materials used in the post-endodontic restoration of root-treated teeth and examines their performance under stress to provide insights for material selection in clinical applications. Particular attention is given to zirconium oxide, which demonstrates promising characteristics due to its esthetic color and favorable material properties, positioning it as a potential material for future use in post-endodontic treatments. Three materials—prefabricated quartz fiber-reinforced composite, milled zirconium oxide, and additively manufactured cobalt–chromium—were evaluated using compressive-deflection tests. The specimens were subjected to a 45° compressive load extending 5 mm from a metal core. Their mechanical properties were analyzed using one-way ANOVA and Tukey's post hoc test. Significant differences were observed among the materials. Quartz fiber posts, with the lowest force resistance, buckled at lower loads (143.3 ± 9.9 N), while zirconia posts failed in a brittle manner at higher forces (246.1 ± 97.2 N). Cobalt–chromium posts demonstrated the highest maximal force (323.2 ± 10.5 N, $p < 0.001$) and, unlike the other materials, bent rather than fractured. The failure patterns of the tested materials underscore the importance of careful material selection when restoring root-treated teeth. Despite displaying distinct fracture characteristics, zirconium oxide, due to its color, rigidity, and hardness, stands out as a promising material for future dental applications. Further research through randomized clinical trials is recommended to refine treatment approaches and optimize clinical outcomes.

Keywords: zirconium oxide; post-endodontic treatment; fracture behavior; quartz fiber posts; root-treated teeth; cobalt–chromium

1. Introduction

Modern post-endodontic materials, such as milled zirconia, provide esthetic benefits. However, compared to other state-of-the-art materials like selective laser-melted cobalt–chromium and glass fiber posts, milled zirconia displays unique properties and distinct fracture behaviors. Understanding these differences aids in making informed decisions when selecting posts for root-treated teeth.

The restoration of endodontically treated teeth often necessitates post core systems, especially when coronal tissue is insufficient for restoration. As an integral part of dental treatment options, post and core restorations hold significant importance in dental prosthetics [1]. They are essential in restoring the structural integrity and ensuring the long-term functionality of teeth, particularly in cases with significant substance loss. The longevity and fracture resistance of the treated teeth depend on the material chosen, the cementing method, and the post's thickness [2,3]. While prefabricated systems, typically comprising quartz fiber or titanium posts, have been in use for some time, severely damaged teeth with minimal remaining tooth structure may require custom-made posts [4]. These are designed to distribute forces optimally, fit perfectly, and leverage the ferrule effect to minimize fracture risks, thus enhancing the tooth's lifespan post-endodontically.

The success of post-endodontic tooth restoration is significantly influenced by the ferrule height and the number of remaining coronal walls [5,6]. These factors are key in reducing stress on the post and the remaining tooth tissue. Traditionally, custom-made cast post cores have been the method of choice for restoring teeth with extensive damage. However, such techniques can be time-consuming and require meticulous execution [7]. Cobalt–chromium alloys are widely recognized as one of the most prominent base metal alloys utilized in dentistry, demonstrating various successful clinical applications. They are characterized by their excellent biocompatibility, high strength, heat resistance, and non-magnetic properties, as well as their ability to resist wear, corrosion, and tarnish. The high modulus of elasticity of cobalt–chromium alloys provides the necessary strength and rigidity for reducing the weight of metal structures [8]. While most of the cobalt–chromium alloys used in the industrial and biomedical fields today originated from the research of Elwood Haynes during the previous century, the techniques used to process this material have since significantly changed [9]. With the appearance of selective laser melting (SLM), achieving predictable results in production, fitting, and material homogeneity has become more feasible. Consequently, this technology is increasingly becoming a part of routine dental restoration procedures [10]. Fiber-reinforced composite posts, introduced in the 1990s, incorporate materials like glass, quartz, or carbon fibers within an epoxy or methacrylate matrix. Their flexibility, dentin-like elasticity modulus, and metal-free composition make them ideal for esthetic applications, particularly in anterior teeth. However, clinical studies suggest a higher failure rate for these posts over ten-years, primarily due to breakage and loss of retention [11]. Contrarily, ceramic materials, particularly zirconium oxide, have been used extensively since 1969 due to their esthetic superiority over metals. Zirconium oxide's high biocompatibility, resistance to corrosion, and chemical stability make it a preferred choice. Despite its brittleness and difficulty in removal or replacement when fractured, zirconium oxide posts demonstrate impressive success rates, with studies indicating a survival probability of over 80% over a decade [12]. The advancements in computer-assisted design and manufacturing (CAD/CAM) technology have revolutionized post and core restorations with ceramic materials, allowing the fabrication of accurately fitting, digitally designed restorations. It is beneficial from an esthetic perspective, where tooth-colored and white posts and cores are favored to avoid color discrepancies with adjacent teeth. Despite the prevalence of these materials, research into the fracture behavior of posts made from cobalt–chromium, zirconium oxide, and quartz fiber remains limited. While studies focus on the clinical performance and long-term success of post-restored teeth, post-fracture issues remain a significant complication in clinical practice. The comparative studies conducted by various researchers provide deeper insights into the performance and suitability of post materials. These studies demonstrate the superiority in mechanical strength of zirconium oxide posts, similar failure rates between fiber-reinforced composite posts and metal posts, and no significant differences in the success and survival rates of glass fiber posts compared with cast metal posts [13–15].

The hypothesis of this study is that there are no significant differences in the mechanical properties of the tested materials. The aim is to determine whether all materials demonstrate comparable characteristics suitable for the restoration of root canal-treated anterior teeth.

2. Materials and Methods

To compare the primary outcome measure with a power of 80% and a significance level of α = 5%, a sample size calculation determined that seven samples per group were needed to detect a difference of 10 percentage points between the groups, assuming a standard deviation of 6%. A 10% change in mechanical properties is considered a clinically meaningful difference. For this reason, ten samples per group were used to investigate the mechanical properties. Three different materials of post-endodontic posts were studied. Initially, ten quartz fiber-reinforced composite posts of ISO size four in green (X-Post, Dentsply Sirona), consisting of 60% quartz fibers and 40% epoxy resin, were reconstructed in the CAD software "Fusion 360 v.2.0.19994" (Autodesk, San Francisco, California, United States). The designs had identical post geometries and were reproduced using computer-aided manufacturing (CAM).

Ten zirconium oxide posts were milled from a zirconium oxide blank (Copran, White-peaks Dental Solutions, Hamminkeln, Germany) using a five-axis milling machine (CORiTEC 150i PRO, imes-icore). The milling process included a lateral support structure, which was later removed and polished.

The metal posts were additively manufactured from a biocompatible cobalt–chromium–tungsten powder (Remanium star CL; Dentaurum) under a nitrogen atmosphere, using a high-power fiber laser (Mlab cusing R; Concept Laser) with a laser power of 56 watts and a scanning speed of 500 mm/s. The layer thickness was set at 30 µm. After fabrication, the posts were sandblasted to achieve a homogenous surface.

A customized testing approach, as described by Lambjerg-Hansen et al. (1997), was selected over a standardized test for evaluating post-endodontically treated teeth because standardized tests generally lack the specificity needed to simulate the clinical environment of these restorations accurately [16]. Post-endodontic teeth have unique structural considerations and stress distributions, often involving weakened areas due to prior treatment. The customized method allows for the measurement of the stiffness, elastic limit, and fracture strength of posts under conditions that closely replicate clinical stresses. This tailored approach provides a more reliable assessment of post durability and stability, thus enhancing its clinical relevance [17].

Mechanical testing was carried out using a tensile testing machine with a maximum force range of 10 kN (Autograph AGS-X Series, Shimadzu, Kyōto, Japan). The sample extended 5 mm from a custom-made metal fixture and was clamped at an angle of 45° (Figure 1a) to the post axis in the testing machine (Figure 1b).

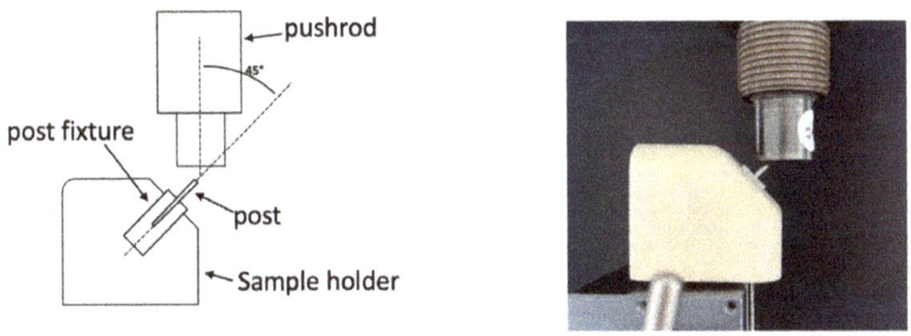

(**a**) (**b**)

Figure 1. Testing machine with custom-made fixture clamping samples at 45° angle—schematic diagram (**a**), experimental setup (**b**).

The sample holder, along with the samples, was aligned and fixed in the screw clamp of the testing machine and pre-set to ensure consistent testing conditions. This setup ensured that an angle of 45° between the post axis and the test body was reproducible for each test. A pushrod of 20 mm in diameter was subjected to a displacement rate of

2 mm/min until the fracture of the sample or maximum displacement of 2.5 mm first occurred. The force and displacement were recorded at 100 Hz. The statistical analysis compared the three materials' stiffness, elasticity limit, and maximum force. A preload of 10 N was applied to ensure the specimen was fully settled in the fixture. This prevented any initial shifting or compliance effects, so that all recorded values accurately represent the material's response.

The stiffness, elastic limit, and maximum force were derived from the force–displacement data obtained from mechanical testing. Stiffness was calculated as the ratio of the applied force to the corresponding displacement within the linear (elastic) region of the force–displacement curve. Specifically, the force at the elastic limit was divided by the maximum elastic displacement in mm at that point. This approach provided a measure of stiffness in N/mm, capturing the material's resistance to elastic deformation. The elastic limit was identified as the point on the force–displacement curve where significant deviation from linearity first occurred, indicating the transition from elastic to plastic behavior. This method allowed us to objectively define the onset of plastic deformation without requiring an offset strain, focusing instead on the visual inflection point where elastic behavior ceased. To assess the load-bearing capacity of each material, the maximum applied force before failure was recorded. Due to the distinct failure behaviors—such as brittle for zirconium oxide, ductile in metal posts, and partial structural breakdown in quartz fibers—this maximum force was selected as a consistent indicator of material performance across varied material types.

The mean and standard deviation for each parameter were calculated and rounded to two decimal places for clarity. An ANOVA test was conducted to compare the three materials, with the significance level set at $p < 0.05$. A Tukey post hoc test was employed to find statistical differences between the materials. All calculations were performed using SPSS Statistics Version 27 (IBM, New York, NY, USA).

The fracture surface and material surfaces of the specimens were observed using a Field-Emission Gun scanning electron microscope (FEG-SEM), Tescan Mira 3 (Tescan, Brno, Czech Republic). Images were acquired at an acceleration voltage of 10 kV using a secondary electron detector. Non-conductive samples were coated with carbon (~10 nm thickness).

3. Results

Tests at 45° showed distinct behaviors among the three tested post materials, as observed in Figure 2. The metal posts exhibited plastic deformation without rupture at the end of the test. Samples of zirconium oxide and quartz fiber groups resulted in a definable fracture. A consistent fracture pattern was observed across the two groups. The fracture line was almost horizontal, perpendicular to the post axis, with no splintering. The quartz fiber-reinforced composite posts bent at a defined maximum load (N), but the fragments remained connected due to undamaged fibers. The fracture line was identifiable by a cloudy-white discoloration, running vertically along the fibers.

Figure 3 shows force–displacement curves for each group, with a representative curve provided for each material. Cobalt–chromium posts reached a plateau in the range of 300–350 N, indicating that these posts reached their maximum load limit without apparent fracture or cracking (Figure 3a). The force–displacement diagrams in Figure 3b revealed visible micro-cracks at low forces in quartz fiber posts. The transition to the plastic phase was not clear, with a prolonged displacement phase and repeated fiber cracking. The diagram in zirconium oxide posts showed a linear increase in force without plastic deformation with typical abrupt failure below 2 mm displacement (Figure 3c).

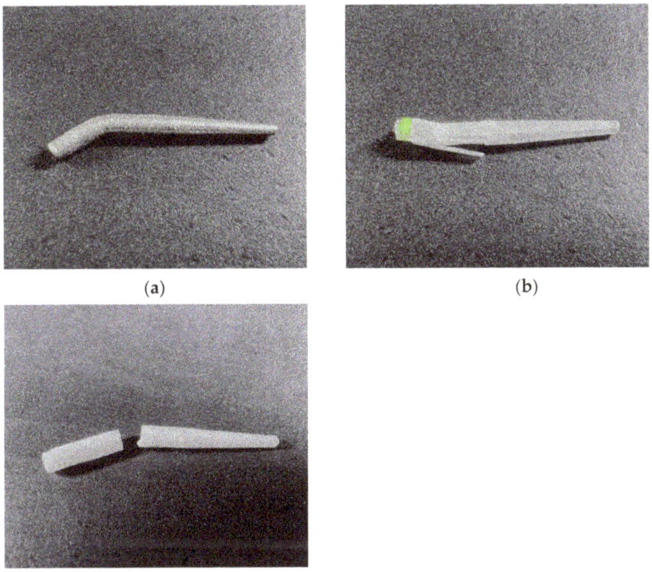

(a) (b) (c)

Figure 2. Samples (posts) after test at 45°: (**a**) cobalt–chromium alloy, (**b**) quartz fiber-reinforced composite, (**c**) zirconium oxide.

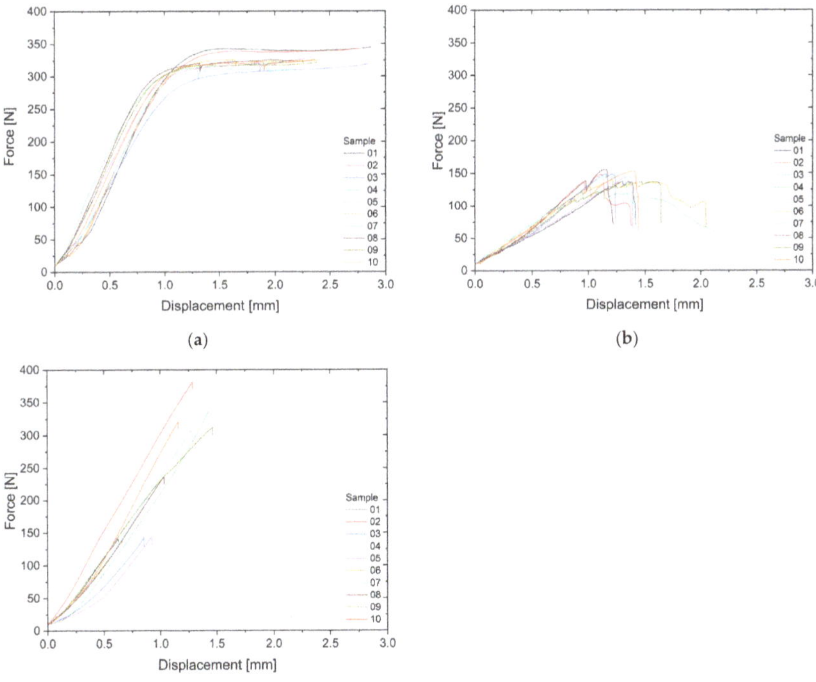

Figure 3. Force–displacement curves depicting group characteristics. (**a**) 10 cobalt-chromium posts, (**b**) 10 quartz fiber posts, (**c**) 10 zirconium oxide posts.

Table 1 summarizes the findings of the three materials. Zirconium oxide posts showed no plastic behavior, with high stiffness (224.5 ± 43.8 N/mm) and maximum force and an elastic limit of 246.1 ± 97.2 N, indicating a lack of ductility.

Table 1. The stiffness, elastic limit, and maximum force of the studied materials.

Parameter	Material	Min	Max	Mean	SD
Maximum force (N)	Cobalt–chromium	310.7	342.3	323.2	10.5
	Quartz fiber	122.3	156.2	143.3	9.9
	Zirconium oxide	137.8	382.1	246.1	97.2
Elastic Limit (N)	Cobalt–chromium	240.0	300.0	273.3	16.9
	Quartz fiber	108.0	141.0	129.8	11.0
	Zirconium oxide	137.8	382.1	246.1	97.2
Stiffness (N/mm)	Cobalt–chromium	272.7	358.9	313.2	28.5
	Quartz fiber	106.2	143.6	126.1	12.2
	Zirconium oxide	154.2	297.6	224.5	43.8

Quartz fiber and cobalt–chromium posts demonstrated lower elastic limit values compared to their maximum force values, indicating some plasticity. Cobalt–chromium posts exhibited the highest maximum force (323.2 ± 10.5 N) without visible damage during testing. In contrast, quartz fiber posts showed the lowest values across all metrics: elastic limit (129.8 ± 11.0 N), maximum force (143.3 ± 9.9 N), and stiffness (162.1 ± 12.2 N/mm). Zirconium oxide posts displayed stiffness values more comparable to cobalt–chromium posts but performed differently under maximum force. A detailed statistical evaluation, including a Tukey post hoc test, is shown in Figure 4. Statistically significant differences were observed in the studied parameters across all three materials. Quartz fiber posts had minimal variation in stiffness values, concentrated between 106.2 N/mm and 143.6 N/mm. Zirconium oxide posts showed the widest range of stiffness values, from 154.2 N/mm to 297.6 N/mm (Table 1, Figure 4a).

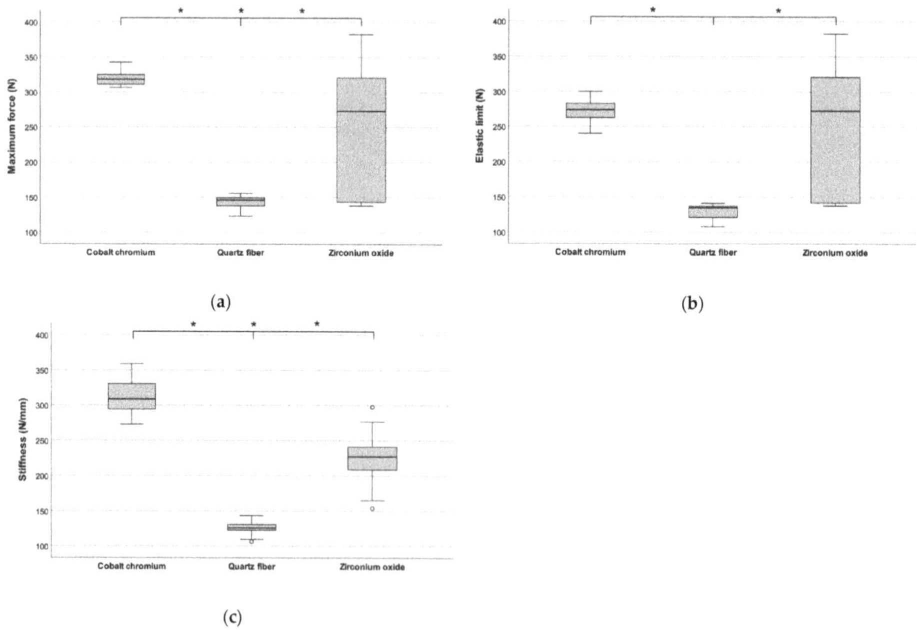

Figure 4. Box plots of tensile testing results. (**a**) Maximum force, (**b**) elastic limit, (**c**) stiffness. Statistically significant results marked with asterisk (*) (n = 10, $p < 0.001$).

Cobalt–chromium posts fell in between, with a stiffness range of 272.7 N to 358.9 N/mm. The elasticity limit of cobalt–chromium posts varied from 240 N to 300 N. Quartz fiber posts had a mean elastic limit of 129.8 N.

The cobalt–chromium posts exhibited the highest maximum force values, with low variation, ranging from 310.7 N to 342.3 N, with a mean value of 323.2 N. In contrast, the zirconium oxide posts showed the largest range, with maximum force values from 137.8 N to 382.1 N and a mean value of 246.1 N.

Figure 5 shows the SEM images of the surfaces of the metal and quartz fiber posts, as well as the fracture surface of the zirconium oxide post. The additively manufactured cobalt–chromium alloy exhibited a crack-free surface with visible printing layers at maximum deflection (Figure 5a), while the quartz fiber posts exhibited mixed damage under the same testing conditions, with observable micro-cracks in the matrix, delamination/debonding, and fiber rupture (Figure 5b). These observations in the quartz fiber posts agree with comparable SEM investigations carried out in three-point tested samples [18]. The zirconium oxide posts demonstrated a clean fracture surface with a homogeneous material structure, free from any porosities (Figure 5c).

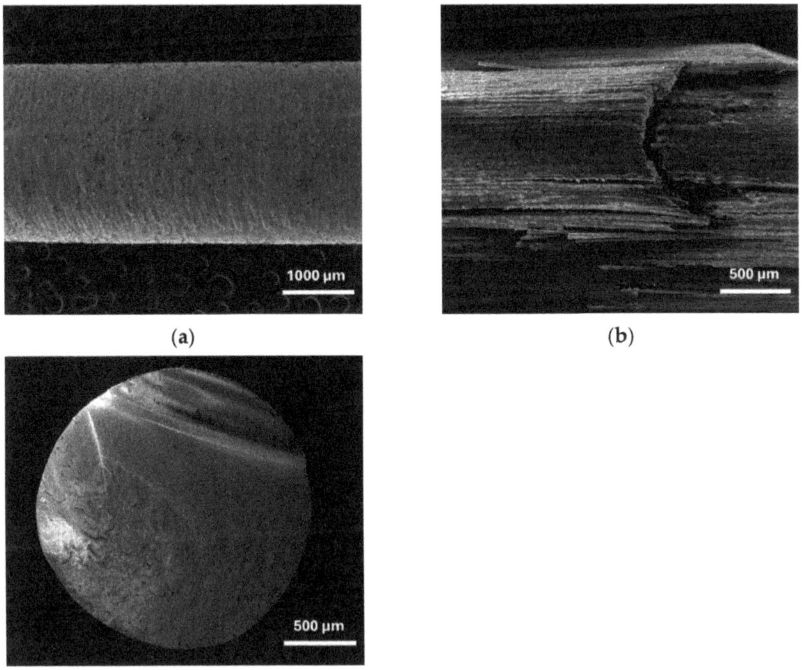

(a) (b) (c)

Figure 5. SEM images at the posts' maximum displacement point: (**a**) Surface of cobalt–chromium alloy. (**b**) Detail of the fracture zone of the quartz fiber post. (**c**) Detail of the fracture surface of the zirconium oxide post.

4. Discussion

The hypothesis of our study, positing no significant differences in the mechanical parameters of the tested materials, can be refuted. The statistical analysis clearly indicated significant variances among the materials, emphasizing the importance of material selection in post-endodontic treatments. Clinical relevance is paramount, especially considering the high occlusal loads that post-endodontic teeth must endure. The focus on compressive-deflection tests under a 45° angled load is particularly relevant, as this angle closely mimics the human interincisal angle and reflects the non-axial nature of masticatory forces in the anterior region. Zirconium oxide posts exhibited a high maximum force (246.1 ± 97.2 N) and stiffness; however, their brittleness was evident due to their limited plastic deformation. The large variance in tensile strength within the zirconium oxide posts group could likely be attributed to the manufacturing process. Manual interventions, such as the removal of lateral support structures during fabrication, may introduce micro-weaknesses, influencing the broad span of force.

Cobalt–chromium posts demonstrated a high maximum force (323.2 ± 10.5 N) without fracturing under pressure. Instead, they deformed, which can be attributed to their low yield strength. These findings confirm their established reliability and effectiveness in clinical settings. Quartz fiber posts, however, were notable for their relatively low maximum force (143.3 ± 9.9 N). The occurrence of micro-cracks at loads as low as 20 N suggests a propensity for fracturing (Figure 5c) under increased loads, even though they are capable of withstanding physiological masticatory forces in the anterior region. This study also shed light on the challenges in the manufacturing processes of these posts. While computer-assisted design and additive manufacturing (selective laser melting) showed efficiency and precision, subtractive manufacturing faced several limitations, particularly in the production of zirconium oxide posts. The issues encountered, such as tool vibrations and the need for manual post-processing, potentially contributed to the variability in the results and highlight the need for further enhancements in manufacturing techniques.

In clinical practice, cost is an important factor influencing material selection. While the initial investment for a cobalt–chromium laser melting device is high, the ongoing costs for cobalt–chromium powder and maintenance are relatively low. This cost structure enables amortization with higher production volumes, making cobalt–chromium posts cost-effective in high-demand settings. On the other hand, quartz fiber posts are industrially manufactured and comprise multiple components, which results in moderately higher costs due to the pricing set by manufacturing companies. Thus, these posts lack the customization potential of cobalt–chromium and zirconium oxide posts, manufactured in dental laboratories. Zirconium oxide posts can be produced using milling machines, with lower initial costs than laser melting devices. Zirconium oxide blanks exhibit high fracture resistance, while the operating costs remain low due to minimal tool wear, as the zirconia reaches its final hardness only after the sintering process.

Comparative studies further underscore the complexity of choosing the right material, highlighting that while some materials may exhibit higher strength, their failure modes and long-term performance under clinical conditions can differ significantly. One study conducted a notable in vitro fracture analysis using 40 extracted human single-rooted premolars [13]. These teeth were subjected to root canal treatments and then categorized into four groups, including one with Zirconium Oxide post core constructions. The testing, involving a 130° angle load until fracture, revealed that the zirconium oxide group exhibited significantly higher fracture resistance (315.4 ± 53.4 N) than all other groups. The lowest test values were observed in the cast metal post core group. Notably, the majority of fractures occurred in the cervical half of the root, rendering them irreparable. This study underscores the superior mechanical strength of zirconium oxide posts, albeit highlighting their vulnerability to catastrophic failure modes.

In another comprehensive investigation, Martins et al. conducted a detailed literature review and meta-analysis comparing fiber-reinforced composite posts and metal posts in endodontically treated teeth [14]. This study included ten research works involving 704 participants and 844 posts. The analysis covered aspects like absolute and relative failure, differentiating between anterior and posterior regions. The conclusion drawn was that there was no significant difference between the posts in terms of survival after failures. However, a limitation of this study was that only six of the included studies had an average evaluation period of more than five years, suggesting the need for longer-term evaluations to fully understand the implications of post material choice.

Another study conducted a fatigue testing study where all specimens were subjected to simultaneous mastication simulation and thermocycling. They found that both the cast metal and zirconia post-and-core groups exhibited similar fatigue resistance, surpassing that of the fiber-reinforced groups. A different approach was taken in another study with a randomized double-blind study, focusing on the success of glass fiber posts versus cast metal post [15]. The study involved human teeth treated endodontically without ferrule, comparing 72 cast metal posts and 111 glass fiber posts, all restored with metal–ceramic crowns. The five-year results indicated no significant differences in success and survival rates between the two materials. However, the study hinted at the necessity of long-term clinical studies to draw more definitive conclusions about long-term success.

These comparative studies, in conjunction with our findings, highlight the complex interplay of factors influencing the choice of post materials in endodontic treatments. While materials like zirconium oxide and cobalt–chromium show high tensile strength, their behavior under load and mode of failure differ significantly from materials like quartz fiber posts, which exhibit lower tensile strength but different failure characteristics. These differences are crucial for clinicians to consider, as the choice of post material can significantly impact the long-term success and functionality of endodontically treated teeth. The variation in study methodologies, angles of load application, and types of failure also demonstrate the need for a standardized approach in evaluating post materials to draw more universally applicable conclusions.

While this study offers valuable insights, a few minor limitations should be noted. The use of a non-standardized testing setup, including loading at a 45° angle rather than in a traditional bending configuration, was chosen to prioritize clinical relevance, though it limits direct comparability to standardized values. Additionally, the manual preparation of samples, particularly for zirconia, may have introduced variability due to potential effects of post-processing on material integrity. A preload of 10 N was necessary to stabilize the fixture, though it may slightly affect measurement precision at the lower end of the force range.

5. Conclusions

Based on the insights gained from this in vitro study, it can be concluded that the tested post materials can withstand the physiological forces encountered in the anterior region of the mouth. Metal posts, long regarded as the standard reference, exhibit clinically desirable mechanical properties but fall short in meeting esthetic requirements. Quartz fiber-reinforced composite posts present a transparent, simple, and cost-effective alternative. The low elastic modulus of the quartz fiber-reinforced composite helps to reduce stress peaks and the incidence of root fractures. However, they are more prone to loosening and damage due to fiber rupture and matrix cracking, as observed in the SEM images.

Modern esthetic post materials like zirconium oxide exhibit excellent mechanical properties. It is concluded that manufacturing identical posts from metals through additive manufacturing or from zirconium oxide through subtractive manufacturing is technically feasible. Moreover, these posts meet the clinical requirements in terms of mechanical properties. However, it is important to note that the workflow for the subtractive manufacturing of longer posts is not yet fully optimized and has room for improvement.

The findings of this study suggest that zirconium oxide could play a significant role in the future, potentially replacing metal-based custom-made posts in clinical practice. Its outstanding mechanical properties and biocompatible nature, as well as its white color, make it a promising candidate for use in dental restorations, especially in anterior regions. Future research should therefore focus more intensively on this material to fully explore its potential and limitations and develop optimal processing and application strategies.

To advance our understanding of post-and-core systems' performance in clinical scenarios, randomized clinical trials incorporating various types of posts—both off-the-shelf and custom-made—are warranted. Such studies could offer valuable insights into the long-term success and durability of different post materials in real-world clinical settings.

Author Contributions: Methodology, A.S. (Armin Sokolowski), F.G.W., B.R. and A.S. (Alwin Sokolowski); Software, B.R.; Validation, F.G.W., B.R. and M.R.; Formal analysis, A.S. (Armin Sokolowski), L.S. and L.K.-B.; Investigation, A.S. (Armin Sokolowski), F.G.W., L.S., L.K.-B. and A.S. (Alwin Sokolowski); Resources, M.R.; Data curation, L.S. and M.R.; Writing—original draft, A.S. (Armin Sokolowski) and L.S.; Writing—review & editing, A.S. (Armin Sokolowski), F.G.W. and A.S. (Alwin Sokolowski); Visualization, F.G.W. and M.R.; Supervision, A.S. (Armin Sokolowski), L.K.-B. and A.S. (Alwin Sokolowski); Project administration, A.S. (Alwin Sokolowski). All authors have read and agreed to the published version of the manuscript.

Funding: This research received no external funding.

Institutional Review Board Statement: Not applicable.

Informed Consent Statement: Not applicable.

Data Availability Statement: The data supporting the findings of this study are available from the corresponding author upon reasonable request.

Acknowledgments: The authors thank Irene Mischak (Department of Dental Medicine and Oral Health, Medical University of Graz, Austria) for her statistical consultation. The authors also thank the laboratory technician Philipp Tepesch (Department of Dental Medicine and Oral Health, Medical University of Graz, Austria) for his exceptional contributions in producing the cobalt–chromium posts, the dental laboratory BananaCAD for the production of the zirconium posts, and Martin Lorenzoni (Former Chair of Division of Restorative Dentistry, Periodontology and Prosthodontics, Medical University of Graz, Austria) for generously providing the necessary infrastructure to support our investigation.

Conflicts of Interest: The authors declare no conflicts of interest.

References

1. Iaculli, F.; Rengo, C.; Lodato, V.; Patini, R.; Spagnuolo, G.; Rengo, S. Fracture Resistance of Endodontically-Treated Maxillary Premolars Restored with Different Type of Posts and Direct Composite Reconstructions: A Systematic Review and Meta-Analysis of in Vitro Studies. *Dent. Mater.* **2021**, *37*, e455–e484. [CrossRef] [PubMed]
2. Alhajj, M.N.; Qi, C.H.; Sayed, M.E.; Johari, Y.; Ariffin, Z. Fracture Resistance of Titanium and Fiber Dental Posts: A Systematic Review and Meta-Analysis. *J. Prosthodont.* **2022**, *31*, 374–384. [CrossRef] [PubMed]
3. Bacchi, A.; Fernandes dos Santos, M.; Pimentel, M.; Caetano, C.; Sinhoreti, M.A.; Consani, R.L. Influence of Post-Thickness and Material on the Fracture Strength of Teeth with Reduced Coronal Structure. *J. Conserv. Dent.* **2013**, *16*, 139. [CrossRef] [PubMed]
4. Veeraganta, S.K.; Samran, A.; Wille, S.; Kern, M. Influence of Post Material, Post Diameter, and Substance Loss on the Fracture Resistance of Endodontically Treated Teeth: A Laboratory Study. *J. Prosthet. Dent.* **2020**, *124*, e1–e739. [CrossRef] [PubMed]
5. Samran, A.; El Bahra, S.; Kern, M. The Influence of Substance Loss and Ferrule Height on the Fracture Resistance of Endodontically Treated Premolars. An in Vitro Study. *Dent. Mater.* **2013**, *29*, 1280–1286. [CrossRef] [PubMed]
6. Dejak, B.; Młotkowski, A. The Influence of Ferrule Effect and Length of Cast and FRC Posts on the Stresses in Anterior Teeth. *Dent. Mater.* **2013**, *29*, e227–e237. [CrossRef] [PubMed]
7. Balkenhol, M.; Wöstmann, B.; Rein, C.; Ferger, P. Survival Time of Cast Post and Cores: A 10-Year Retrospective Study. *J. Dent.* **2007**, *35*, 50–58. [CrossRef] [PubMed]
8. Evans, E.J.; Thomas, I.T. The in Vitro Toxicity of Cobalt-Chrome-Molybdenum Alloy and Its Constituent Metals. *Biomaterials* **1986**, *7*, 25–29. [CrossRef] [PubMed]
9. Al Jabbari, Y.S. Physico-Mechanical Properties and Prosthodontic Applications of Co-Cr Dental Alloys: A Review of the Literature. *J. Adv. Prosthodont.* **2014**, *6*, 138. [CrossRef] [PubMed]
10. van Noort, R. The Future of Dental Devices Is Digital. *Dent. Mater.* **2012**, *28*, 3–12. [CrossRef] [PubMed]
11. Naumann, M.; Koelpin, M.; Beuer, F.; Meyer-Lueckel, H. 10-Year Survival Evaluation for Glass-Fiber-Supported Postendodontic Restoration: A Prospective Observational Clinical Study. *J. Endod.* **2012**, *38*, 432–435. [CrossRef] [PubMed]
12. Bateli, M.; Kern, M.; Wolkewitz, M.; Strub, J.R.; Att, W. A Retrospective Evaluation of Teeth Restored with Zirconia Ceramic Posts: 10-Year Results. *Clin. Oral. Investig.* **2014**, *18*, 1181–1187. [CrossRef] [PubMed]
13. Kalyoncuoğlu, E.; Ural, Ç.; Aydemir, H.; Aslan, M.A.; Balkaya, V. Effect of 1-Piece Post and Core Fabrication Techniques on Fracture Strength. *J. Appl. Biomater. Funct. Mater.* **2015**, *13*, 253–258. [CrossRef] [PubMed]
14. Martins, M.D.; Junqueira, R.B.; de Carvalho, R.F.; Lacerda, M.F.L.S.; Faé, D.S.; Lemos, C.A.A. Is a Fiber Post Better than a Metal Post for the Restoration of Endodontically Treated Teeth? A Systematic Review and Meta-Analysis. *J. Dent.* **2021**, *112*, 103750. [CrossRef] [PubMed]
15. Sarkis-Onofre, R.; Amaral Pinheiro, H.; Poletto-Neto, V.; Bergoli, C.D.; Cenci, M.S.; Pereira-Cenci, T. Randomized Controlled Trial Comparing Glass Fiber Posts and Cast Metal Posts. *J. Dent.* **2020**, *96*, 103334. [CrossRef] [PubMed]

16. Lambjerg-Hansen, H.; Asmussen, E. Mechanical Properties of Endodontic Posts. *J. Oral. Rehabil.* **1997**, *24*, 882–887. [CrossRef] [PubMed]
17. Asmussen, E.; Peutzfeldt, A.; Heitmann, T. Stiffness, Elastic Limit, and Strength of Newer Types of Endodontic Posts. *J. Dent.* **1999**, *27*, 275–278. [CrossRef] [PubMed]
18. Lo Giudice, G.; Cagidiaco, E.F.; Lo Giudice, R.; Puleio, F.; Nicita, F.; Calapaj, M. Evaluation of Mechanical Properties of a Hollow Endodontic Post by Three Point Test and SEM Analysis: A Pilot Study. *Materials* **2019**, *12*, 1983. [CrossRef] [PubMed]

materials

MDPI

Article

Visibility of Recurrent Caries Through Universal Shade Resin Composite Restorations

Ryotaro Yago [1,*,†], Chiharu Kawamoto [1,*,†], Di Wu [2], Takuma Mirokuin [1], Rafiqul Islam [2], Monica Yamauti [3], Hidehiko Sano [2] and Atsushi Tomokiyo [2]

1 Department of Restorative Dentistry, Graduate School of Dental Medicine, Hokkaido University, Kita 13 Nishi 7, Kita-ku, Sapporo 060-8586, Japan; adjmtw9165@gmail.com
2 Department of Restorative Dentistry, Faculty of Dental Medicine, Hokkaido University, Kita 13 Nishi 7, Kita-ku, Sapporo 060-8586, Japan; wudi0526@den.hokudai.ac.jp (D.W.)
3 Department of Biomedical and Applied Science, School of Dentistry, Indiana University, 1121 W. Michigan St., Indianapolis, IN 46202, USA; myamauti@gmail.com
* Correspondence: ryago@den.hokudai.ac.jp (R.Y.); chipa@den.hokudai.ac.jp (C.K.); Tel.: +81-11-706-4261 (R.Y. & C.K.)
† These authors contributed equally to this work.

Abstract: This in vitro study aimed to investigate whether color differences in the stained cavity floor simulating recurrent caries can be detected using various restored resin composites. Artificial teeth were made with conventional resin composite (Estellite Sigma Quick A3; ET), and class V cavities were prepared. To simulate the color of caries, a dot was marked in the center of the cavity floor using four different magic pens. The cavities were filled with ET and two universal shade resin composites (UC, Omnichroma; OMI, Essentia Universal; ESS). For photographic analysis, a standard correction color chart was used. The color difference (ΔE_{00}) between (i) the lab value at the center of the cavity and (ii) the average lab value at 1 mm mesial and distal to the center of the cavity was calculated. The data were statistically analyzed using two-way ANOVA ($p < 0.05$). For visual analysis, 25 dentists were asked to complete a questionnaire to determine whether the color differences were noticeable. In the photographic analysis, UC showed larger ΔE_{00} values than ET in all colors. Visual analysis revealed higher detection rates for UC than ET. Universal shade resin composite tends to reflect the color of the cavity more effectively than conventional resin composite.

Keywords: recurrent caries; caries detection; resin composite; universal shade resin composite; structural color

1. Introduction

In recent years, resin composites have been used extensively because of their improved mechanical strength and bond strength, as well as their excellent esthetic qualities [1–3]. However, in some clinical situations, recurrent caries (secondary caries) may occur but not break away, delaying the detection of caries in some cases.

According to a Japanese government report, more than 90% of adults in Japan have experienced dental caries in the past, 30% of adults have untreated dental caries, and dental caries is the cause of approximately 40% of tooth extractions in people over 40 years old [4]. One of the characteristics of adult dental caries is recurrent caries [5]. Recurrent caries is more likely to progress deeper into the dentin and is therefore more likely to lead to pulpitis [6]. The government cautions that pulp-treated teeth are less likely to be painless, further delaying the detection of caries [6].

Recurrent caries is usually detected through visual and radiographic examinations [7–10]. Early detection of recurrent caries allows minimal intervention and the conservation of more tooth structures [11]. In the case of recurrent caries under a resin composite, if patients can look at their teeth in a mirror and notice changes, it is expected to trigger a visit to the dentist, leading to early detection and treatment. It may also lead to an improvement in the sensitivity of dentists' visual examination.

Dental caries can be classified into acute and chronic caries [12]. Acute caries is more common in young people, while chronic caries is more common in middle-aged and older adults [13]. The color of softened dentin in acute caries is pale yellow, whereas that in chronic caries is brown to blackish brown [14].

In recent years, universal shade resin composite (UC) has been developed to match the color of teeth with a single paste [15,16]. They are based on structural color [17] or light-scattering properties [18]. Conventional resin composites (non-UC) achieve a good color match with the tooth structure by adding pigments [17,19,20].

Omnichroma (OMI) is a UC based on structural color that develops by selectively interacting with the nanostructure of the tooth [17]. The uniform spacing and arrangement of spherical OMI particles facilitates the transmission of light throughout the restoration [21]. It reflects the color of the cavity surrounding the restoration and obtains a color match through blending [22].

Essentia Universal (ESS) is a microhybrid UC with a blending effect [23]. The light transmission and scattering properties of ESS with microhybrid fillers are known to blend naturally with the surrounding tooth structure [24].

Estellite Sigma Quick (ET) is a non-UC and contains pigment.

When targeting the color of caries, the use of natural teeth would make evaluation between materials difficult due to the large variation in color. Therefore, we used a method to determine the detection ability of caries color under uniform color conditions using magic pens and resin composites.

The purpose of this study was to simulate artificial caries in a standardized class 5 cavity using a magic pen and filling it with UC and non-UC and (1) to measure the color difference after filling (2) to conduct a questionnaire survey to dentists to determine if the color difference was obvious by visual examination.

The null hypotheses are (1) there is no color difference due to the difference in the color given, (2) there is no color difference due to the difference in the material, and (3) the difference in the material affects the detection rate due to the difference in the operator.

2. Materials and Methods

2.1. Preparation of Specimens

The materials used in the study are listed in Table 1. In this study, ET (A3 shade, Tokuyama Dental, Tokyo, Japan) was used as the conventional resin composite, and OMI (Tokuyama Dental) and ESS (GC, Tokyo, Japan) were used as the UCs. The specimen preparation procedure is shown in Figure 1. A standard cavity of 2.5 mm in length, 3.5 mm in width, and 2.0 mm in depth in an artificial tooth (A5A-500, Nissin, Kyoto, Japan) was prepared using a diamond (FG 401, Shofu, Kyoto, Japan). A replica impression was made using silicon material (Memodil 2, Kulzer, Hanau, Germany). The surface of the impression was filled with ET and then irradiated for 40 s using a light irradiator (Pencure 2000, Morita, Tokyo, Japan; irradiation intensity 2000 mW/cm^2).

Table 1. Materials used in this study.

Material (Code)	Filler Type (Percent per Weight)	Composition	Percent per Weight	Manufacturer	Lot
Estelite Sigma Quick A3 (ET)	Supra-nano spherical filler (82)	2-Propenoic Acid, 2-Methyl-, (1-Methylethylidene) Bis [4,1- Phenyleneoxy (2-Hydroxy-3,1-Propanediyl)] Ester	10–30	Tokuyama Dental, Tokyo, Japan	J3051
		Triethylene Glycol Dimethacrylate	5–10		
		2,6-Di-tert-Butyl-p-Cresol	<1		
		p-Methoxyphenol	<1		
		Titanium Dioxide	<0.1		

Table 1. *Cont.*

Material (Code)	Filler Type (Percent per Weight)	Composition	Percent per Weight	Manufacturer	Lot
Omnichroma (OMI)	Supra-nano spherical filler (79)	7,7,9(or7,9,9)-Trimethyl-4,13-Dioxo-3,14-Dioxa-5,12-Diazahexadecane-1,16-Diyl Bismethacrylate	10–30	Tokuyama Dental	019E89
		2,2′-Ethylenedioxydiethyl Dimethacrylate	1–5		
		2,6-Di-tert-Butyl-p-Cresol	<1		
		Dl-Bornane-2,3-Dione	<1		
		Mequinol	<1		
Essentia Universal (ESS)	Microhybrid filler (81)	Urethane Dimethacrylate	10–25	GC, Tokyo, Japan	2003091
		Ytterbium Trifluoride	5–10		
		(Octahydro-4,7-Methano-1H-Indenediyl) Bis (methylene) Bismethacrylate	2.5–5		
		2-(2H-benzotriazol-2-yl)-p-cresol	0.1–0.2		

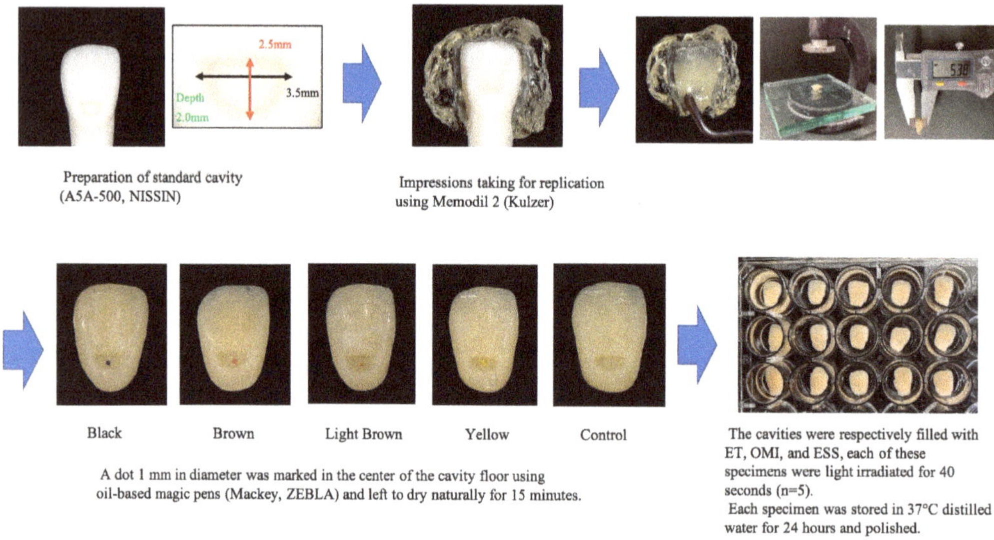

Figure 1. Sample preparation procedures of the specimens.

To simulate caries color, a dot (approximately 1 mm) in diameter was marked at the center of the cavity floor with four color (black, brown, light brown, and yellow) oil-based magic pens (Mackey, Zebla, Tokyo, Japan) and left to dry for 15 min. To standardize the location of the dots, the center of the cavity was determined with a stereomicroscope when coloration was applied. The cavities were incrementally filled with ET, OMI, or ESS without adhesive application and irradiated with light for 40 s. For the control group, resin teeth without markings were prepared. Each sample was stored in distilled water at 37 °C for 24 h. The specimens were polished with a silicon point (White Point CA, Shofu) and a soft polisher (Super Snap, Shofu) for 30 s each and stored in water. The specimens from each group (n = 5) are shown in Figure 2.

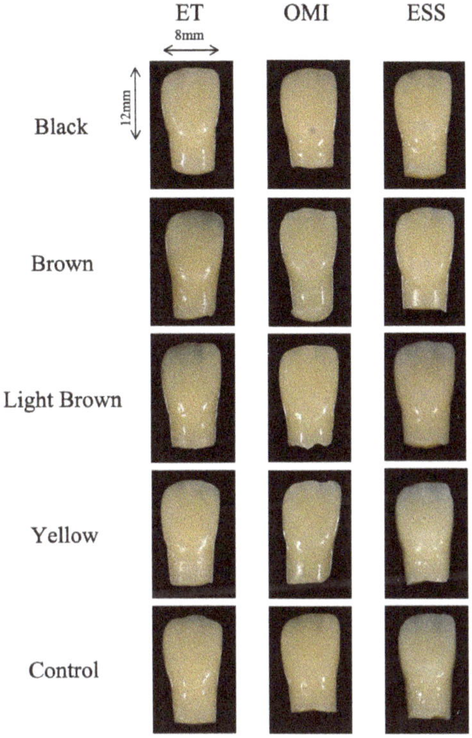

Figure 2. Specimens of each group after polishing.

2.2. Photographic Analysis

Photographic analysis was performed using image-corrected color cards (CASMATCH, Bearmedic, Ibaraki, Japan). Photographic conditions included a darkroom, a shooting distance of 100 mm, and a black background. Representative images are shown in Figure 3 panel (1). Image editing software (Adobe Photoshop 2021, Adobe, San Jose, CA, USA) was used for image analysis. To calibrate the color of the image, the sampling range of the eyedropper tool was adjusted to the average of a 5 × 5 pixels square. Correcting contrast and gray balance by setting reference values for color level correction produces images with consistent tone levels. *CIE L*a*b** and CIEDE 2000 color difference formulas were used for color evaluation [25,26]. *CIE L*a*b** values were recorded at the center of the cavity and at points 1 mm mesial and distal to the center of the cavity (Figure 3 panel (2)). To eliminate bias due to measurement points, each sample was measured three times and the average value was used as the data. The color difference (ΔE_{00}) between (i) the lab value at the center of the cavity and (ii) the average lab value at 1 mm mesial and distal to the center of the cavity was calculated using the CIEDE 2000 Formula (1).

$$\Delta E_{00} = \left[\left(\frac{\Delta L'}{k\mathrm{LSL}}\right)2 + \left(\frac{\Delta C'}{k\mathrm{CSC}}\right)2 + \left(\frac{\Delta H'}{k\mathrm{HSH}}\right)2 + \mathrm{RT}\left(\frac{\Delta C'}{k\mathrm{LSC}}\right)\left(\frac{\Delta H'}{k\mathrm{HSH}}\right)\right]^{1/2} \quad (1)$$

2.3. Visual Analysis

For visual analyses, one sample was randomly selected from each group to form three irregularly arranged plates. A total of 25 dentists and 25 volunteers were included in the study. The 25 licensed dentists were not less than 24 years of age, had less than 40 years of post-graduation experience, had bilateral naked eye visual acuity $\geq$ 0.6 or corrected visual acuity $\geq$ 0.8, and were free of color blindness or strong color deficiencies. The details are shown in Tables A1–A3 (Appendix A). The 25 volunteers had to be at least 20 years old, with bilateral naked eye visual acuity ≥ 0.6 or corrected visual acuity ≥ 0.8, and without color blindness or strong color weakness, and not be a licensed dentist, dental hygienist, or dental technician. The details are shown in Tables A4 and A5. The test was conducted in a double-blind manner. Each sample was visually inspected for significant color differences. First, the subjects were shown an unfilled control sample. They were then shown the plates and asked to judge within 2 s for each sample whether "the color difference is noticeable" or "do not know, cannot judge", and to fill out the questionnaire. Finally, they were asked to vote for the sample with the most noticeable color difference in each plate.

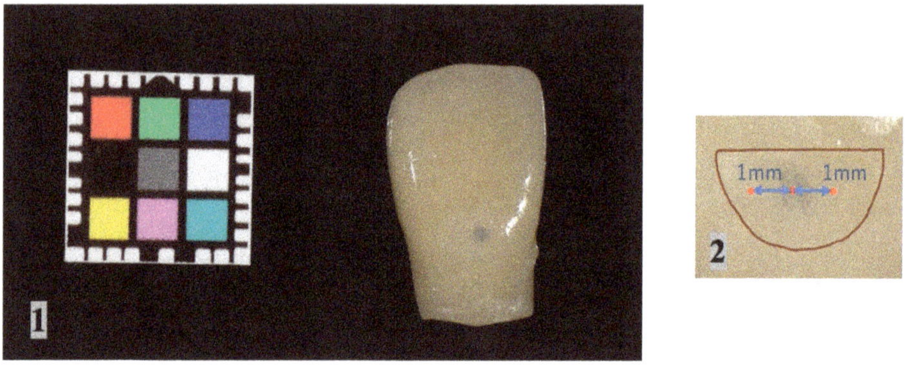

Figure 3. Photographic analysis. **1**: Photographed using Casmatch. **2**: *CIE L*a*b** was recorded at the center of the cavity and 1 mm mesial and distal to the center of the cavity.

2.4. Statistical Analysis

Two-way ANOVA was used to examine the effects of three different materials and five different colors (including the control) on ΔE_{00}. When the interaction was significant, Bonferroni's method was used to examine the simple main effect at each factor level. The Bonferroni method was used for post-hoc tests. SPSS ver. 29.0 (IBM, Armonk, NY, USA) was used for statistical analysis, with a significance level of 5%.

3. Results

Figure 4 shows for every group of photographic data the mean and standard deviation of ΔE_{00}. The three materials and the five colors (including the control) exhibited a substantial interaction in the two-way ANOVA [F (8, 74) = 122.19, $p < 0.001$]. The Bonferroni method investigates straightforward main effects at each factor level. The ET group did not exhibit any significant differences among the five colors, including the control. All categories in the ESS group exhibited a significant difference ($p < 0.01$), except between the Brown and Black groups. Among the ET, OMI, and ESS groups, the control group exhibited no significant differences.

Figure 5 shows the estimated peripheral averages of ΔE_{00}. The graph indicates that the trend of ΔE_{00} among the five colors varied among materials. There appears to be a difference between the colors in OMI and ESS, except between the Black and Brown in ESS. However, there was less distinction between the five colors in the ET. The ΔE_{00} difference between the five colors of the three materials indicates interaction. The graph shows that Black, Brown, Light Brown, and Yellow had the same data pattern of ET < ESS < OMI, but the control did not have a distinct trend. The interaction effect refers to the difference in ET, ESS, and OMI between the five colors (including the control).

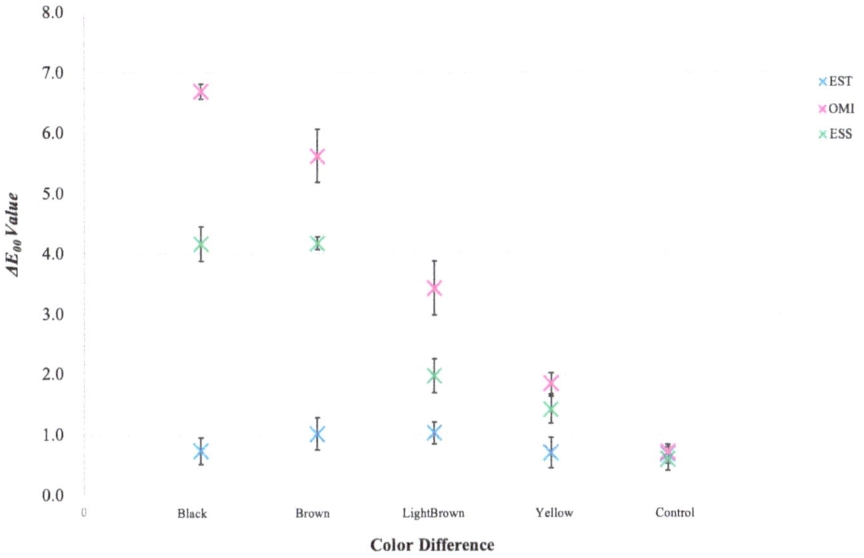

Figure 4. The mean and standard deviation of ΔE_{00} for each group of photographic analysis data. Two-way analysis of variance revealed a significant interaction between the three materials and the five colors (F (8, 74) = 122.19, $p < 0.001$). The Bonferroni method was used to examine the simple main effect for each level of each factor, and no significant differences were found between the five colors in the ET. In the OMI, there were significant differences among all five colors ($p < 0.001$), and in the ESS, there were significant differences among all groups, except between Brown and Black ($p < 0.01$). No significant differences were found between the ET, OMI, and ESS groups and the control group.

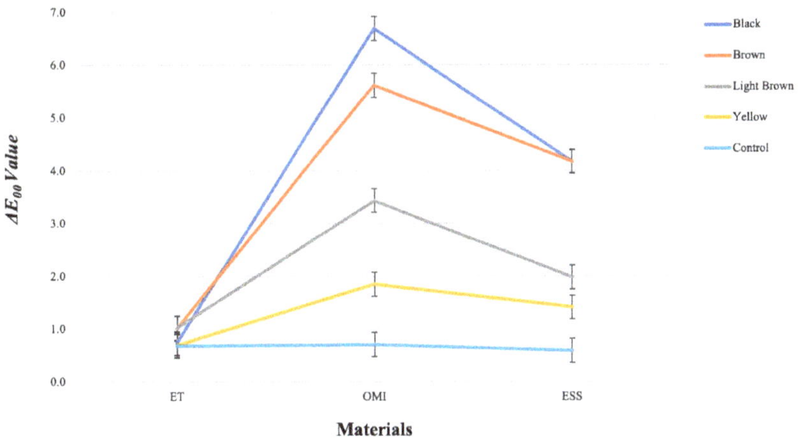

Figure 5. Estimated marginal means of ΔE_{00}. Error bar: 95% CI. The trend of ΔE_{00} among the five colors of the materials is different, and there appears to be a difference between the colors in OMI and ESS, except between Black–Brown in ESS. However, it can be seen that there is less difference between the five colors in ET. This difference in the ΔE_{00} trends among the five colors of the three materials indicates an interaction. The graph also shows that Black, Brown, Light Brown, and Yellow have the same data trend of ET < ESS < OMI, while Control does not show such a clear trend. Thus, the difference in the trends of ET, ESS, and OMI among the five colors indicates the meaning of the interaction effect.

Visual analysis was conducted with 25 licensed dentists and 25 volunteers, each evaluating three trays containing 15 different types of randomly arranged samples. Each subject made 45 individual judgments. Tables 2 and 3 present the data in a tabular format, detailing the percentages of "noticeable" and "non-noticeable" judgments. Among the materials analyzed, Black exhibited the highest proportion of "noticeable" judgments, with Brown, Light Brown, and Yellow following in a descending sequence. This was the same trend for both dentists and volunteers. Results for dentists showed that the ESS group was 99% Black, 79% Brown, and 59% Light Brown, revealing a difference of over 20% when compared to the OMI group's Brown and Light Brown categories. The ET group's Black percentage was 72%, indicating a divergence from the figures reported by OMI and ESS. ET was 72% for Black, a difference of more than 20% between OMI and ESS. Conversely, the differences between the materials were less than 10% for Yellow, 3% for ET, 1% for OMI, and 8% for ESS. In addition, 8% of the Control samples were judged "noticeable" by ET, 4% by OMI, and 3% by ESS.

Table 2. Percentage of "noticeable" calculated from visual analysis results [1].

		Black	Brown	Light Brown	Yellow	Control
Dentist	ET	72	47	23	3	8
	OMI	99	97	93	1	4
	ESS	99	79	59	8	3
Volunteer	ET	72	29	27	4	15
	OMI	100	77	60	5	12
	ESS	96	49	36	11	11

[1] Values in the table are in percent (%).

Table 3. Percentage of "not noticeable" calculated from visual analysis for dentists results [1].

		Black	Brown	Light Brown	Yellow	Control
Dentist	ET	28	53	77	97	92
	OMI	1	3	7	99	96
	ESS	1	21	41	92	97
Volunteer	ET	28	71	73	96	85
	OMI	0	23	40	95	88
	ESS	4	51	64	89	89

[1] Values in the table are in percent (%).

Three plates were prepared for visual analysis, each with one sample from each of the 15 groups (3 materials × 5 colors). The judges comprised 25 licensed dentists and 25 volunteers. Out of these three plates, they chose the one with the most noticeable color difference. A total of 75 votes, with 3 votes each for each of the 25 participants. The voting results are presented in Tables 4 and 5. OMI–Black received the most votes among dentists (58/75), followed by ESS–Black (12/75), OMI–Light Brown (3/75), OMI–Brown (1/75), and ET–Black (1/75). OMI–Black received the most votes among volunteers (42/75), followed by ESS–Black (28/75), OMI–Brown (2/75), ET–Black (2/75) and OMI–Light Brown (1/75).

Table 4. Voting results of the visual analysis for dentists.

Rank	Material	Color	Votes
1st	OMI	Black	58
2nd	ESS	Black	12
3rd	OMI	Light Brown	3
4th	OMI	Brown	1
5th	ET	Black	1

Table 5. Voting results of visual analysis for volunteers.

Rank	Material	Color	Votes
1st	OMI	Black	42
2nd	ESS	Black	28
3rd	OMI	Brown	2
4th	ET	Black	2
5th	OMI	Light Brown	1

4. Discussion

Resin composites are widely used in anterior and molar tooth because of dentin adhesive [27–31]. However, in clinical situations, recurrent caries may occur but not break away, delaying the detection of caries in some cases. Patients identify recurrent caries through color change, symptoms, and fissures, potentially postponing treatment.

Various composite resin products have been developed for different applications [1–3]. Recently, UC has garnered recognition as a single-shade resin that offers excellent color compatibility with teeth of diverse shades [15,16]. The first UC product, Omnichroma, was released in 2020, followed by Essensia Universal, ClearFill Majesty ES Flow Universal (Kuraray Noritake), and Beautiful Unishade (Shofu) [15–17,20,32,33]. Because UC is influenced by the color of the surrounding area, patients who can glance in the mirror and see changes in their teeth when recurring caries arise should anticipate seeing their dentist for early detection and treatment. Since UC is affected by the surrounding color, if patients can look at their teeth in a mirror and notice changes when recurrent caries occurs, it is expected to trigger a visit to the dentist, leading to early detection and early treatment.

In this study, several types of magic pens were prepared to simulate caries and composite resin was used instead of teeth. Usually, natural teeth are used in these experiments. However, the use of natural teeth is likely to result in large variations in dentin color, making evaluation between materials difficult. Therefore, we used a method of determining the visibility concerning the color of caries under conditions of uniform color using a magic pen and resin composite.

The color of caries differs between acute and chronic caries, with the softened dentin of acute caries being light yellow, whereas the softened dentin of chronic caries is brown to blackish brown [14]. Therefore, four different colors were used in this study.

Common spectrophotometers possess a minimum measurement range of 3 to 5 mm in diameter, which complicates the prediction of narrow regions. In this study, we used the image correction marker Casmatch (5 × 5 pixels range) for measurements.

CIEDE 2000 color difference formula was published in 2001 and is frequently used in dentistry to evaluate color differences, which was also used in this study [24,34–38].

The results of the photographic analysis showed significant differences between materials among almost all colors in the UC, but no significant differences among groups, including the Control, in EST of conventional resin composite. In addition, comparisons between colors showed identical data trends such as EST < ESS < OMI for Black, Brown, Light Brown, and Yellow, but no such clear trend was observed for the controls. This is the meaning of the interaction. Therefore, the null hypotheses (1) there is no color difference due to the color given and (2) there is no color difference due to material differences are rejected. Therefore, it can be said that the conventional resin composite did not affect the visualization of the cavity floor and the cavity floor may be visible in UC restorations. This may be because conventional resin composite achieves a good color match with the dentin by adding pigments [17,19,20], whereas UC blends naturally with tooth by reflecting or diffusing the surrounding color due to properties such as structural color [17] and light scattering [18].

For each color, OMI showed significant differences in all groups, while ESS showed significant differences in all groups except between Brown and Black, indicating different trends in results among the UCs.

Omnichroma is a UC based on structural color that develops by selectively interacting with the nanostructure of the tooth [17]. The uniform spacing and arrangement of spherical OMI particles facilitates the transmission of light throughout the restoration [21]. It reflects the color of the cavity surrounding the restoration and obtains a color match through blending [22].

Essentia Universal is a microhybrid UC with a blending effect [23]. The light transmission and scattering properties of ESS with microhybrid fillers are known to blend naturally with the surrounding tooth structure [24].

A previous study comparing the light transmittance characteristics of OMI and ESS found that ESS has a wider light transmission intensity distribution and better diffusion behavior than OMI [23]. Composite resins such as ESS have light diffusion properties that obscure the boundary with the surrounding tooth [39], whereas OMI has light diffusion and low opacity [22]. It is assumed that these differences in optical properties influenced the differences in results between the UCs.

The visual analysis included 25 licensed dentists and 25 volunteers who were not licensed dentists, dental hygienists, or dental technicians, with bilateral naked eye visual acuity of 0.6 or better or corrected visual acuity of 0.8 or better, and without color blindness or strong color weakness.

As in the photographic analysis, there is a high proportion of Black and Brown and a low proportion of Light Brown and Yellow. Especially in the case of Yellow, where almost all materials are in the same single-digit range, the color can be difficult to notice. Trends in the photographic analyses were similar to those in the visual analyses. Therefore, the null hypothesis of (3) the difference in the material affects the detection rate due to the difference in the operator was rejected. Regardless of the operator, UC tended to judge color differences as significant, at least for dark colors such as Black and Brown. This was the same trend for both dentists and volunteers.

Based on the above, UC restorations may be useful in detecting recurrent caries that may occur in the future. An individualized approach is recommended for adult caries, including secondary caries [5]. However, it is important for patients to be aware of recurrent caries and to visit a dentist, regardless of whether they choose to follow-up or to have restorations.

5. Conclusions

Within the limits of this study, the following can be concluded: Universal shade resin composite tends to reflect the color of the cavity more effectively than ordinary composite resins. Moreover, this is particularly applicable to structural color types compared to light-scattering types. Using universal shade resin composites makes it easier to detect color changes in cavities, perhaps leading to early identification of recurring caries with color changes.

Author Contributions: Conceptualization, R.Y. and C.K.; methodology, R.Y., C.K. and R.I.; software, D.W.; validation, T.M., R.I. and M.Y.; formal analysis, R.Y., H.S. and A.T.; investigation, R.Y., T.M. and D.W.; resources, M.Y. and A.T.; data curation, R.Y., C.K. and T.M.; writing—original draft preparation, R.Y., C.K., D.W., T.M., M.Y. and A.T.; writing—review and editing, R.Y., C.K., R.I., H.S. and A.T.; visualization, R.Y., C.K. and D.W.; supervision, H.S.; project administration, C.K.; funding acquisition, R.Y., C.K. and H.S. All authors have read and agreed to the published version of the manuscript.

Funding: This study was supported by JST SPRING, Grant Number JPMJSP2119.

Institutional Review Board Statement: The questionnaire survey conducted in this study was not applicable for research that requires ethical review under the Ethical Guidelines for Medical and Health Research Involving Human Subjects established by the Japanese government (Ministry of Health, Labour and Welfare).

Informed Consent Statement: Informed consent was obtained from all subjects involved in this study.

Data Availability Statement: The data presented in this study are available on request from the corresponding author due to privacy.

Conflicts of Interest: The authors declare no conflicts of interest.

Appendix A

A total of 25 licensed dentists who were at least 24 years old, less than 40 years post-dental school, with bilateral naked eye visual acuity ≥ 0.6 or corrected visual acuity ≥ 0.8, and without color blindness or strong color weakness were included in the study. The distributions of participants' gender, age, and clinical experience are shown in Tables A1–A3.

Table A1. Gender Distribution of the Participants (Dentists).

	Male	**Female**
Number	13	12

Table A2. Clinical Experience Distribution of the Participants (Dentists).

	Resident (<1 Y)	**Grad Student (1–5 Y)**	**Junior Faculty [1]**	**Senior Faculty [2]**
Number	7	8	4	6

[1] Instructor class less than 10 years after graduation. [2] Instructor class more than 10 years after graduation.

Table A3. Age Distribution of the Participants (Dentists).

	20 s	**30 s**	**40 s**	**50 s**
Number	13	6	2	4

A total of 25 volunteers who were at least 20 years old, with bilateral naked eye visual acuity ≥ 0.6 or corrected visual acuity ≥ 0.8, and without color blindness or strong color weakness, and were not licensed as dentists, dental hygienists, or dental technicians were included in the study. The distributions of participants' gender and age are shown in Tables A4 and A5.

Table A4. Gender Distribution of the Participants (Volunteers).

	Male	**Female**
Number	17	8

Table A5. Age Distribution of the Participants (Volunteers).

	20 s	**30 s**	**40 s**	**50 s**	**60 s**	**70 s**
Number	14	4	2	2	2	1

References

1. Fusayama, T. The process and results of revolution in dental caries treatment. *Int. Dent. J.* **1997**, *47*, 157–166. [CrossRef] [PubMed]
2. Ferracane, J.L. Resin composite—State of the art. *Dent. Mater.* **2011**, *27*, 29–38. [CrossRef] [PubMed]
3. Rajabi, H.; Denny, M.; Karagiannopoulos, K.; Petridis, H. Comparison of Flexural Strength and Wear of Injectable, Flowable and Paste Composite Resins. *Materials* **2024**, *17*, 4749. [CrossRef] [PubMed]
4. Ministry of Health Labour and Welfare, Japan. Survey of Dental Diseases. 2016. Available online: https://www.mhlw.go.jp/toukei/list/62-28.html (accessed on 17 October 2024).
5. Schwendicke, F.; Splieth, C.H.; Bottenberg, P.; Breschi, L.; Campus, G.; Doméjean, S.; Ekstrand, K.; Giacaman, R.A.; Haak, R.; Hannig, M.; et al. How to intervene in the caries process in adults: Proximal and secondary caries? An EFCD-ORCA-DGZ expert Delphi consensus statement. *Clin. Oral Investig.* **2020**, *24*, 3315–3321. [CrossRef]
6. Ministry of Health Labour and Welfare, Japan. Characteristics and Prevalence of Caries in Adults. Available online: https://www.e-healthnet.mhlw.go.jp/information/teeth/h-02-003.html (accessed on 17 October 2024).
7. Brouwer, F.; Askar, H.; Paris, S.; Schwendicke, F. Detecting Secondary Caries Lesions: A Systematic Review and Meta-analysis. *J. Dent. Res.* **2016**, *95*, 143–151. [CrossRef]
8. Mjör, I.A. Clinical diagnosis of recurrent caries. *J. Am. Dent. Assoc.* **2005**, *136*, 1426–1433. [CrossRef]

9. Schwendicke, F.; Brouwer, F.; Paris, S.; Stolpe, M. Detecting Proximal Secondary Caries Lesions: A Cost-effectiveness Analysis. *J. Dent. Res.* **2016**, *95*, 152–159. [CrossRef]
10. Lino, J.R.; Ramos-Jorge, J.; Coelho, V.S.; Ramos-Jorge, M.L.; Moysés, M.R.; Ribeiro, J.C. Association and comparison between visual inspection and bitewing radiography for the detection of recurrent dental caries under restorations. *Int. Dent. J.* **2015**, *65*, 178–181. [CrossRef]
11. Askar, H.; Krois, J.; Göstemeyer, G.; Bottenberg, P.; Zero, D.; Banerjee, A.; Schwendicke, F. Secondary caries: What is it, and how it can be controlled, detected, and managed? *Clin. Oral Investig.* **2020**, *24*, 1869–1876. [CrossRef]
12. Fusayama, T.; Okuse, K.; Hosoda, H. Relationship between Hardness, Discoloration, and Microbial Invasion in Carious Dentin. *J. Dent. Res.* **1966**, *45*, 1033–1046. [CrossRef]
13. Theodore, M.R.; Clifford, M.S.; Roger, E.B.; Joe, T.W. Fundamentals in cavity preparation. In *The Art and Science of Operative Dentistry*, 3rd ed.; Clifford, M.S., Theodore, M.R., Harald, P.H., John, R.S., Eds.; Mosby: St. Louis, MO, USA, 1995; pp. 289–324.
14. Cheng, L.; Zhang, L.; Yue, L.; Ling, J.; Fan, M.; Yang, D.; Huang, Z.; Niu, Y.; Liu, J.; Zhao, J.; et al. Expert consensus on dental caries management. *Int. J. Oral Sci.* **2022**, *14*, 17. [CrossRef] [PubMed]
15. Lucena, C.; Ruiz-López, J.; Pulgar, R.; Della Bona, A.; Pérez, M.M. Optical behavior of one-shaded resin-based composites. *Dent. Mater.* **2021**, *37*, 840–848. [CrossRef] [PubMed]
16. Ersöz, B.; Karaoğlanoğlu, S.; Oktay, E.A.; Aydin, N. Resistance of Single-shade Composites to Discoloration. *Oper. Dent.* **2022**, *47*, 686–692. [CrossRef] [PubMed]
17. Saegusa, M.; Kurokawa, H.; Takahashi, N.; Takamizawa, T.; Ishii, R.; Shiratsuchi, K.; Miyazaki, M. Evaluation of Color-matching Ability of a Structural Colored Resin Composite. *Oper. Dent.* **2021**, *46*, 306–315. [CrossRef] [PubMed]
18. Murata, T.; Kumagai, T. Light scattering property of composite resin "Essentia". In Proceedings of the 145th Meeting of the Japanese Society of Conservative Dentistry, Nagano, Japan, 27–28 October 2016.
19. Dias, F.A.; Conto, M.V.R.; Guiraldo, R.D.; Geha, O.; Paloco, E.A.C.; Fernandes, T.M.F.; Berger, S.B. Does Pigment Incorporation into Regular Composite Resins for Posterior Buildups Alter Their Bond Strength? *Braz. Dent. J.* **2020**, *31*, 440–444. [CrossRef]
20. Hayashi, K.; Kurokawa, H.; Saegusa, M.; Aoki, R.; Takamizawa, T.; Kamimoto, A.; Miyazaki, M. Influence of surface roughness of universal shade resin composites on color adjustment potential. *Dent. Mater. J.* **2023**, *42*, 676–682. [CrossRef]
21. Pereira Sanchez, N.; Powers, J.M.; Paravina, R.D. Instrumental and visual evaluation of the color adjustment potential of resin composites. *J. Esthet. Restor. Dent.* **2019**, *31*, 465–470. [CrossRef]
22. Kobayashi, S.; Nakajima, M.; Furusawa, K.; Tichy, A.; Hosaka, K.; Tagami, J. Color adjustment potential of single-shade resin composite to various-shade human teeth: Effect of structural color phenomenon. *Dent. Mater. J.* **2021**, *40*, 1033–1040. [CrossRef]
23. Korkut, B.; Özcan, M. Longevity of Direct Resin Composite Restorations in Maxillary Anterior Crown Fractures: A 4-year Clinical Evaluation. *Oper. Dent.* **2022**, *47*, 138–148. [CrossRef]
24. Chen, F.; Toida, Y.; Islam, R.; Alam, A.; Chowdhury, A.; Yamauti, M.; Sano, H. Evaluation of shade matching of a novel supra-nano filled esthetic resin composite employing structural color using simplified simulated clinical cavities. *J. Esthet. Restor. Dent.* **2021**, *33*, 874–883. [CrossRef]
25. *ISO/CIE 11664-4:2019*; Colorimetry—Part 4: CIE 1976 L*a*b* Colour Space. ISO: Geneva, Switzerland, 2019.
26. *ISO/CIE 11664-6:2022*; Colorimetry—Part 6: CIEDE2000 Colour-Difference Formula. ISO: Geneva, Switzerland, 2022.
27. Fusayama, T. Posterior adhesive composite resin: A historic review. *J. Prosthet. Dent.* **1990**, *64*, 534–538. [CrossRef] [PubMed]
28. Worthington, H.V.; Khangura, S.; Seal, K.; Mierzwinski-Urban, M.; Veitz-Keenan, A.; Sahrmann, P.; Schmidlin, P.R.; Davis, D.; Iheozor-Ejiofor, Z.; Rasines Alcaraz, M.G. Direct composite resin fillings versus amalgam fillings for permanent posterior teeth. *Cochrane Database Syst. Rev.* **2021**, *8*, CD005620. [CrossRef] [PubMed]
29. Heintze, S.D.; Ilie, N.; Hickel, R.; Reis, A.; Loguercio, A.; Rousson, V. Laboratory mechanical parameters of composite resins and their relation to fractures and wear in clinical trials-A systematic review. *Dent. Mater.* **2017**, *33*, e101–e114. [CrossRef]
30. Ástvaldsdóttir, Á.; Dagerhamn, J.; van Dijken, J.W.; Naimi-Akbar, A.; Sandborgh-Englund, G.; Tranæus, S.; Nilsson, M. Longevity of posterior resin composite restorations in adults—A systematic review. *J. Dent.* **2015**, *43*, 934–954. [CrossRef]
31. Chan, K.H.S.; Mai, Y.; Kim, H.; Tong, K.C.T.; Ng, D.; Hsiao, J.C.M. Review: Resin Composite Filling. *Materials* **2010**, *3*, 1228–1243. [CrossRef]
32. Maesako, M.; Kishimoto, T.; Tomoda, S.; Horie, T.; Yamada, M.; Iwawaki, R.; Odagiri, Y.; Sakuma, K.; Inoue, K.; Takeguchi, A.; et al. Evaluation of the Repolished Surface Properties of a Resin Composite Employing Structural Coloration Technology. *Materials* **2021**, *14*, 7280. [CrossRef]
33. ClearFill Majesty ES Flow Universal. Available online: https://www.kuraraynoritake.jp/feature/majesty_esflow_universal/ (accessed on 17 October 2024).
34. Luo, M.R.; Cui, G.; Rigg, B. The development of the CIE 2000 colour-difference formula: CIEDE2000. *Color Res. Appl.* **2001**, *26*, 340–350. [CrossRef]
35. Gómez-Polo, C.; Portillo Muñoz, M.; Lorenzo Luengo, M.C.; Vicente, P.; Galindo, P.; Martín Casado, A.M. Comparison of the CIELab and CIEDE2000. color difference formulas. *J. Prosthet. Dent.* **2016**, *115*, 65–70. [CrossRef]
36. Chen, F.; Wu, D.; Islam, R.; Toida, Y.; Kawamoto, C.; Yamauti, M.; Sano, H. Evaluation of Color and Spectral Behavior of a Novel Flowable Resin Composite after Water Aging: An In Vitro Study. *Materials* **2022**, *15*, 4102. [CrossRef]
37. Paolone, G.; Mazzitelli, C.; Boggio, F.; Breschi, L.; Vichi, A.; Gherlone, E.; Cantatore, G. Effect of Different Artificial Staining Proce-dures on the Color Stability and Translucency of a Nano-Hybrid Resin-Based Composite. *Materials* **2023**, *16*, 2336. [CrossRef]

38. Sulaiman, T.A.; Rodgers, B.; Suliman, A.A.; Johnston, W.M. Color and translucency stability of contemporary resin-based restora-tive materials. *J. Esthet. Restor. Dent.* **2021**, *33*, 899–905. [CrossRef] [PubMed]
39. Tsubone, M.; Nakajima, M.; Hosaka, K.; Foxton, R.M.; Tagami, J. Color shifting at the border of resin composite restorations in human tooth cavity. *Dent. Mater.* **2012**, *28*, 81. [CrossRef]

materials

MDPI

Article

Evaluation of Shade Integration of a Novel Universal-Shade Flowable Bulk-Filling Resin Composite

Hirofumi Kaneko [1,†], Chiharu Kawamoto [1,*,†], Yu Toida [1], Ryotaro Yago [1], Di Wu [2], Yuan Yuan [2], Fei Chen [3], Monica Yamauti [4], Hidehiko Sano [2] and Atsushi Tomokiyo [2]

1 Department of Restorative Dentistry, Graduate School of Dental Medicine, Hokkaido University, Kita 13 Nishi 7, Kita-ku, Sapporo 060-8586, Japan; k.cat.hiro5629@den.hokudai.ac.jp (H.K.); ryago@den.hokudai.ac.jp (R.Y.)
2 Department of Restorative Dentistry, Faculty of Dental Medicine, Hokkaido University, Kita 13 Nishi 7, Kita-ku, Sapporo 060-8586, Japan; wudi0526@den.hokudai.ac.jp (D.W.)
3 Department of Stomatology, Beijing Tongren Hospital, Capital Medical University, No. 1, Dongjiaomingxiang Avenue, Dongcheng District, Beijing 100730, China
4 Department of Biomedical and Applied Science, School of Dentistry, Indiana University, 1121 W. Michigan St., Indianapolis, IN 46202, USA
* Correspondence: chipa@den.hokudai.ac.jp; Tel.: +81-11-706-4261
† These authors contributed equally to this work.

Abstract: Background: This study aimed to evaluate the color-matching and light transmission properties of a newly developed aesthetic flowable resin composite, OCFB-001. Methods: Rubber molds containing cylindrical cavities were filled with Estelite Sigma Quick, and 40 resin composite (CR) molds with simulated Class I cavities were prepared in shades A1, A2, A3, and A4, resulting in a total of 160 samples. Following bonding procedures, four different flowable resin composites (n = 10) were introduced into the cavities. The color difference (ΔE_{00}) was calculated using two methods. A two-way analysis of variance was performed, and the interaction was significant, so a post hoc analysis was performed for each shade using Bonferroni's correction. The morphology of the filler in each material was observed via scanning electron microscopy (SEM). Results: In the A1 shade, OCFB-001 demonstrated color differences comparable to those of other materials. However, in the A2, A3, and A4 shades, OCFB-001 exhibited significantly lower color differences (ΔE_{00}) than the other materials, with a more consistent distribution. SEM analysis revealed that the OCFB-001 structure resembled that of Estelite Bulk Fill Flowable. Conclusions: OCFB-001 showed excellent shade matching in the A2, A3, and A4 ranges and good matching in the A1 shade, on par with existing universal-shade flowable bulk-fill resin composites.

Keywords: CIEDE2000; color chart for image correction; colorimeter; SEM; simulated Class I cavity; structural color

1. Introduction

The advancement of adhesive dentistry, coupled with increasing aesthetic demands from patients, has established resin composites as the foremost restorative material in contemporary dental practice [1]. In dental restorative treatment, aesthetic requirements must be met by restoring the anatomy of the tooth and matching the color of the tooth and restorative material [2]. Natural teeth vary in transparency and shade between enamel and dentin and layering techniques have been used to achieve esthetic restorations [3–5]. However, layering techniques require the use of multiple types of resin composites of different shades. In addition, dental shade matching is most commonly performed subjectively by visual selection, which is dependent on the clinician's experience, age, and physical condition [6]. These processes are complex and contribute to increased treatment times.

Universal-shade resin composites have recently emerged, attracting significant interest from clinicians due to their ability to match nearly all tooth shades, thereby simplifying restorative procedures [7].

The aesthetic success of these resin composites, particularly regarding the color tone compatibility with restored teeth, is intrinsically linked to their optical properties. These properties include light transmission, surface reflection, diffusion, absorption, and scattering [8,9]. The type and content of inorganic fillers and organic matrices further influence these optical properties, impacting the chromatic compatibility of the resin composites [10].

Conventional light-cured resin composites usually had to be placed at a thickness not exceeding 2 mm, due to the fact that the light intensity decreases below 2 mm from the surface layer, significantly reducing the depth of cure [11,12]. Therefore, in the case of restorative procedures for deep cavities, the resin composite had to be light-cured many times at a thickness of less than 2 mm, causing a prolonged treatment time. The introduction of bulk-fill resin composites, capable of filling cavities up to 4 mm in depth in a single increment, has significantly reduced treatment times compared to the traditional incremental filling technique [13].

In recent years, universal-shade resin composites have gained significant attention for their versatility in clinical applications [14]. These materials are engineered to match a wide range of tooth shades using a single shade, offering practical advantages in restorative dentistry. Notably, Omnichroma emerged as the first commercially available pigment-free universal-shade resin, utilizing structural coloration through 260 nm spherical fillers that enhance the reflection and refraction of specific light wavelengths [15]. Filler systems that combine spherical filler geometry with reduced average filler size are generally considered to have lower mechanical properties and increased susceptibility to age-related degradation, while filler systems incorporating spherical particles have been reported to lead to improved light transmission [16]. In addition, single-shade resin composites, such as Omnichroma, have an acceptable color-adjustment potential (CAP) [17,18]. This underlines how the concept of one-shade resin composites can be realized in a variety of ways and adds to the diversity found in the field of direct dental restorations [17,18].

Building on this foundational technology, a novel esthetic flowable resin composite, OCFB-001 (OCFB), has been developed.

Our previous research confirmed the excellent color adaptability of Omnichroma resin composite in a simulated 2 mm Class I cavity, supporting its effectiveness for universal-shade applications [19]. More recently, we have demonstrated that Omnichroma Flow also exhibits high color compatibility, characterized by relatively uniform reflectance and enhanced light transmission properties [20].

It has been reported that lightness decreases with the increasing cavity depth [21]. This phenomenon may be more pronounced in non-pigmented universal-shade resins. The esthetic performance of these materials may also be correlated with optical properties. In addition, most of the research reports on color differences of universal-shade resin are within 2 mm depth of cure, and there are few reports on color differences when bulk-fill type universal-shade resin is filled in deep cavities.

Thus, this study aims to assess the color compatibility and optical transmission characteristics of OCFB by fabricating a standardized 4 mm Class I cavity. The null hypothesis was that no significant differences in color compatibility and color parameters would be observed among the universal-shade flowable bulk-fill composite resins tested.

2. Materials and Methods

2.1. Specimen Preparation and Evaluation of Shade Matching

The details of the resin composites used in this study are shown in Table 1.

Table 1. Resin composites, their manufacturers, organic matrices, presence of pigments, and Lot numbers.

	Resin Composites (Code) (Manufactures)	Organic Matrices	Pigments	Lot Numbers
Filling Resin Composites	OCFB-001 (OCFB) (Tokuyama Dental, Tokyo, Japan)	UDMA TEGDMA	-	21102
	Filtek Bulk Fill Flowable (FiBF) (3M ESPE, St. Paul, MN, USA)	Bis-GMA UDMA Bis-EMA (6)	+	NF34174
	SDR flow+ (SDR) (Dentsply Sirona, Charlotte, NC, USA)	TEGDMA EBPADMA	+	2205000974
	Estelite Bulk Fill Flowable (EsBF) (Tokuyama Dental, Tokyo, Japan)	Bis-GMA Bis-MPEPP TEGDMA	+	8228
Mold	Estelite Sigma Quick (ESQ) (Tokuyama Dental, Tokyo, Japan)	Bis-GMA TEGDMA	+	175082

UDMA, urethane dimethacrylate; TEGDMA, triethylene glycol dimethacrylate; Bis-GMA, bisphenol A-glycidyl methacrylate; Bis-EMA (6), bisphenol A-ethoxylated dimethacrylate; EBPADMA, ethoxylated bisphenol A-dimethacrylate; Bis-MPEPP, 2,2′-bis(4-methacryloxyate polyethoxyphenyl)propane.

A 5 mm-thick, 10 mm-diameter acrylic block (Resin Disk Clear, Yamahachi Dental MFG., Co., Aichi, Japan) was used as the base material. The block was processed using a computer-aided design/computer-aided manufacturing (CAD/CAM) system (Ceramill mind, Amann Girrbach GmbH, Pforzheim, Germany) to create a cylindrical cavity with a diameter of 4 mm and a depth of 4 mm. The cutting process was performed using a CAD system in combination with a CAM machine (Ceramill motion2, Amann Girrbach GmbH, Pforzheim, Germany). A polymethyl methacrylate (PMMA) disc was utilized for this procedure, and three types of rotary cutting bars were employed: 0.6 mm diameter (Roto RFID 0.6 DMB DC, Amann Girrbach GmbH, Pforzheim, Germany), 1.0 mm diameter (Roto RFID 1.0 DMB DC, Amann Girrbach GmbH, Pforzheim, Germany), and 2.5 mm diameter (Roto RFID 2.5 DMB DC, Amann Girrbach GmbH, Pforzheim, Germany).

To replicate a simulated Class I cavity, silicone impression material (Sildefit wash type, Shofu Inc., Kyoto, Japan) was used to create a rubber mold from the acrylic block. The mold was designed to have a round cavity with a diameter of 10 mm and a height of 5 mm, as well as a central cylindrical projection matching the cavity dimensions (4 mm diameter and 4 mm depth). The impressions were made with the acrylic block positioned so that the cavity faced upward during the molding process (Figure 1A,B). The silicone mold was allowed to cure and was subsequently stored at room temperature in an incubator for 24 h to ensure complete reaction and to mitigate any potential hydrogen gas release during curing (Figure 1C). Using these molds, 160 frames were created in shades A1, A2, A3, and A4 (n = 40 per shades) by filling the molds with ESQ resin composite. The ESQ resin was light-cured with a light-emitted diode (LED) curing unit (PenCure 2000, Morita, Tokyo, Japan) at an intensity range of 660 to 760 mW/cm^2 [19,20,22] (Figure 1D). As ESQ is not a bulk-fill-type resin, laminate filling was carried out at least twice with a thickness not exceeding 2 mm. The resin composition was slightly overfilled, and the surface was flattened under pressure with a transparent matrix and a glass slide and light-cured.

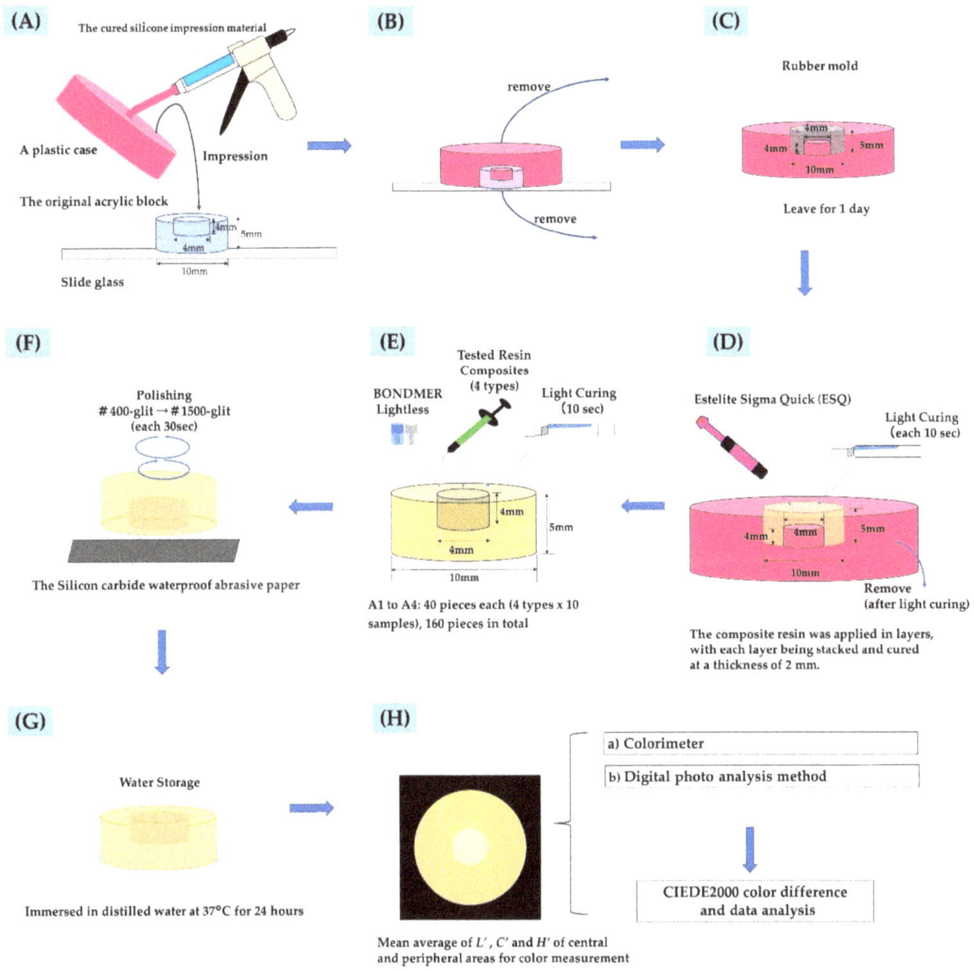

Figure 1. Diagrammatic representation of the specimen preparation for color measurement. The original acrylic block was placed on a glass slide with the cavity facing upward, filled with silicone impression material in a plastic case, and impressions were taken (**A**). A plastic case, the original acrylic block and slide glass were removed (**B**). The silicone mold was stored at room temperature in an incubator for 24 h to ensure complete reaction and to mitigate any potential hydrogen gas release (**C**). Using rubber molds, 160 frames were created in shades A1, A2, A3, and A4 (n = 40 per shades) by filling the molds with ESQ resin composite. The ESQ resin composite was light-cured with an LED curing unit (**D**). These cavities with ESQ framing were treated with a chemical-cure adhesive. Then, four types of resin composites were used to fill the simulated cavities (n = 10 per type).The four resin composites were filled in batches and light-cured for 10 s using an LED curing unit at an intensity of 1470 mW/cm^2 (**E**). The surfaces of the restorations were polished with 400- and 1500-grit silicon carbide waterproof abrasive paper for 30 s (**F**). The polished specimens were stored in distilled water at 37 °C for 24 h (**G**). The Lab values were measured by two different methods and the color difference was calculated. Colorimetry was performed by two methods: (a) colorimetry using a colorimeter, and (b) an intraoral camera was used to capture images of specimens with color- and size-matching stickers placed on color reference tiles, which were then measured using image-processing software (digital photo analysis method) (**H**).

To simulate Class I cavities formed by the cylindrical projections, mock cavities (4 mm in diameter and 4 mm in height) were prepared for each shade, totaling 40 cavities per shade. These cavities were treated with a chemical-cure adhesive (Bondmer Lightless, Tokuyama Dental, Tokyo, Japan) according to the manufacturer's instructions (Figure 1E).

Following surface treatment, four types of resin composites were used to fill the simulated cavities (n = 10 per type; Figure 1E). As with the ESQ framing, the resin composites were slightly overfilled and the surfaces were flattened by pressure with a transparent matrix and glass slides. The four resin composites were filled in batches and light-cured for 10 s using an LED curing unit (Elipar DeepCure-L, 3M ESPE, St. Paul, MN, USA) at an intensity of 1470 mW/cm^2. After light curing, the surfaces of the restorations were polished with 400- and 1500-grit silicon carbide waterproof abrasive paper (Sankyo-Rikagaku Co., Ltd., Saitama, Japan) for 30 s (Figure 1F). The polished specimens were then stored in distilled water at 37 °C for 24 h (Figure 1G).

Colorimetry was performed by two methods: (i) colorimetry using a colorimeter, and (ii) an intraoral camera was used to capture images of specimens with color- and size-matching stickers (CASMATCH, BEAR Medic, Tokyo, Japan) placed on color reference tiles, which were then measured using image-processing software (digital photo analysis method).

(i) Colorimeter measurement

Lab values of the specimens were measured using a colorimeter (OFC-300, RC500, PaPaLaB Co., Tokyo, Japan) under a D65 light source (LDA9N-D-G, TOSHIBA, Tokyo, Japan) [14,15,19]. A color checker (ColorChecker, X-Rite INC., Tokyo, Japan) was used for calibration. The instrument was calibrated with a white background (L^* = 93.2, a^* = −0.3, b^* = −1.6) and a black background (L^* = 0.5, a^* = 0.7, b^* = −0.6) before each series of measurements (Figure 1H-a). Calibration was performed by first capturing the black background over the entire image display area, followed by capturing the white background over the entire image display area.

The illumination geometry employed for the reflectance measurements was bidirectional at 45°/0°. The following figures show the photographic conditions and the dimensional range of the measurement area for the colorimeter measurements (Figures 2 and 3). The shooting distance was 75 mm.

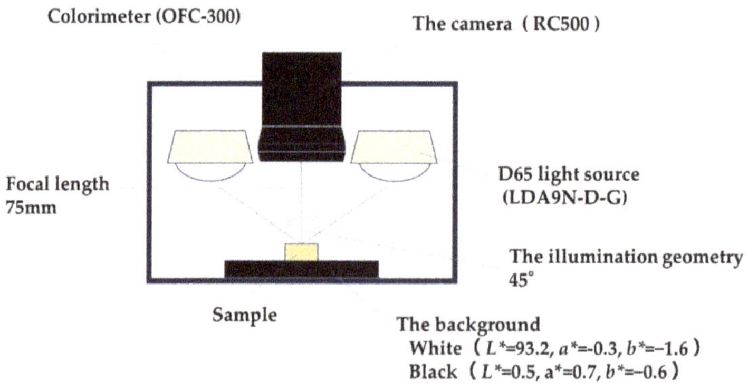

Figure 2. Photographic conditions (colorimeter).

To evaluate the color parameters, the measurement spot should be selected at least 0.3 mm away from the margin, avoiding the intersection between the four filled and framed resin composites [19,20,22]. Therefore, the center of the sample was selected for the filling area and the midpoint between the margin and the edge for the frame area. A circular region of image (ROI; width = 64 pixels (0.809 mm) and distance = 64 pixels (0.811 mm)) was used for colorimetry, and the average of Lab values at 64 locations in the region was calculated.

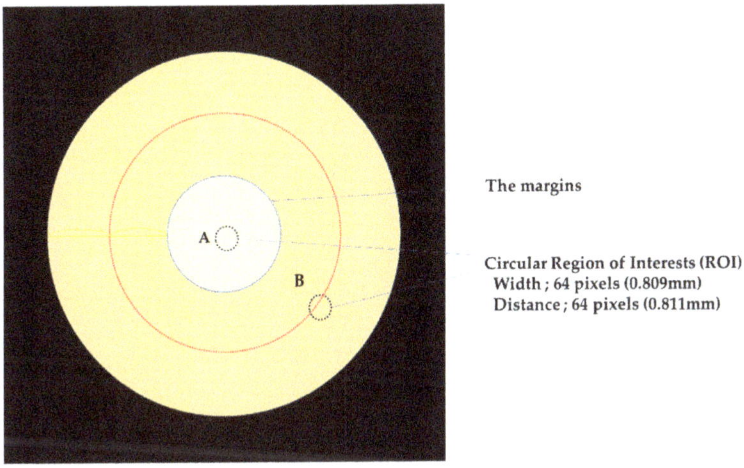

Figure 3. Measurement area dimensions (colorimeter). The measurement spot should be selected at least 0.3 mm away from the margin, avoiding the intersection between the four filled and framed resin composites. The four filled resin composites tested and the center of the sample were selected (A). The Frame resin composites, the midpoint between the margin and the edge were selected (B).

(ii) Digital photo analysis method

An intraoral camera (EyeSpecial C- II, Shofu Inc., Kyoto, Japan) was employed to obtain images of the specimens, along with color- and size-matching stickers (CASMATCH, BEAR Medic, Tokyo, Japan) placed on color reference tiles. The following figures show the photographic conditions and the dimensional range of the measurement area in the digital photo analysis method (Figures 4 and 5). The images were captured under a D65 light source (T-TESOLA, TRUSCO, Tokyo, Japan), which approximates standard daylight conditions. The illumination geometry employed for the reflectance measurements was bidirectional at 45°/0°. Both a white tile (CM-101W, Konica Minolta, Tokyo, Japan) and a black tile (CM-101B, Konica Minolta) were utilized for reference. Photographs were taken using the camera's low-glare mode to minimize surface reflections. The shooting distance was 80 mm.

Lab color values were extracted from the images using Adobe Photoshop (version 7.0, Adobe Inc., San Jose, CA, USA; Figure 1H-b). The color tiles used had Lab values of white background (L^* = 93.56, a^* = −1.97, b^* = 3.53) and black background (L^* = 29.38, a^* = −0.93, b^* = 0.07). Color correction of the images was performed in accordance with the guidelines provided in the CASMATCH correction manual to ensure accurate color representation. The measurement spot was selected at the center of the sample for the filling area and halfway between the margin and the edge for the frame area. Colorimetry was performed three times for both the center and the periphery of each sample, and the average value was calculated. The distance between each point was set to be 1 mm apart and recorded.

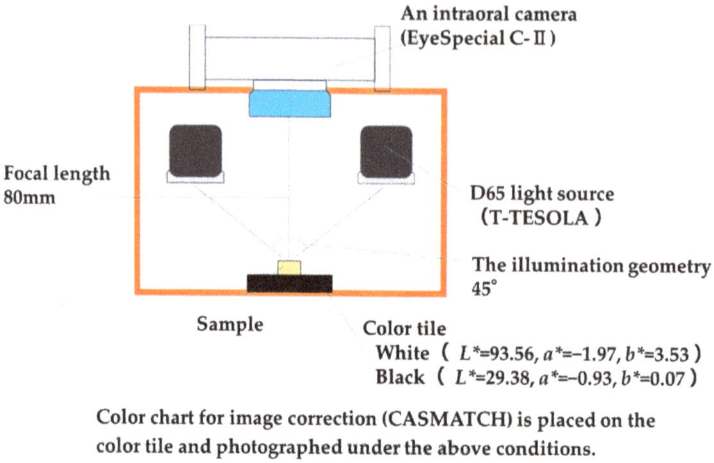

Figure 4. Photographic conditions (digital photo analysis method).

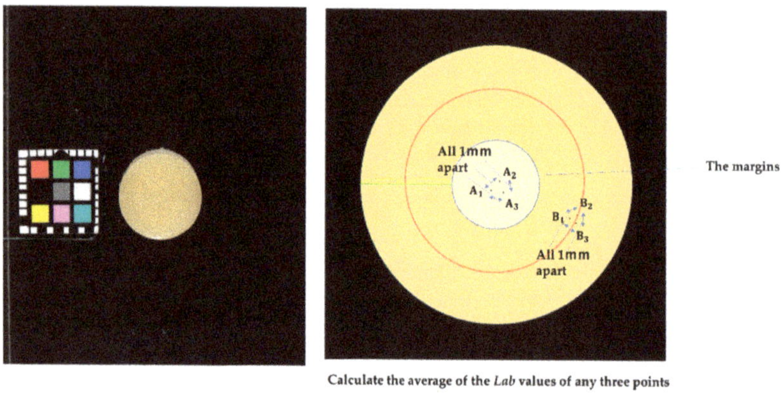

Figure 5. The typical image with color chart and measurement area dimensions (digital photo analysis method). The measurement spot should be selected at least 0.3 mm away from the margin, avoiding the intersection between the four filled and framed resin composites.

The CIE currently recommends using CIEDE2000, which utilizes the concepts of saturation and hue, and the color difference (ΔE_{00}) is calculated using the following formula [23,24]. The ΔE_{00} was calculated using an Excel spreadsheet for calculating CIEDE2000 [25]:

$$\Delta E_{00} = \left[\left(\frac{\Delta L'}{K_L S_L} \right)^2 + \left(\frac{\Delta C'}{K_C S_C} \right)^2 + \left(\frac{\Delta H'}{K_H S_H} \right)^2 + R_T \left(\frac{\Delta C'}{K_C S_C} \right) \left(\frac{\Delta H'}{K_H S_H} \right) \right]^{1/2} \tag{1}$$

where: $\Delta L' = \left[L_{peripheral} - L_{Central} \right]$, $\Delta C' = \left[C_{peripheral} - C_{central} \right]$, $\Delta H' = \left[H_{peripheral} - H_{central} \right]$, R_T is a rotation function that accounts for the interaction between chroma and hue differences, while the weighting functions S_L, S_C, and S_H adjust the total color difference for variations in the location of the color difference. The parametric factors K_L, K_C, and K_H are proposed to control the magnitude of tolerance judgments and adjust for scaling of acceptability rather than perceptibility. Previous research indicates that texture only affects lightness tolerances but not chroma or hue tolerances; therefore, a value of K_L = 2 was proposed [20,24]. The perceptibility threshold (PT) and acceptability threshold (AT) are critical parameters for assessing the color matching of materials in esthetic dentistry [26,27]. Numerous studies have investigated the PT and AT for color differences (ΔE_{ab} and ΔE_{00}) within this field [28,29]. Based on these findings, the 50:50% PT in the CIELAB color space has been established at ΔE_{ab} = 1.2, while the 50:50% AT has been reported as ΔE_{ab} = 2.7 [30,31]. Corresponding values in the CIEDE2000 color difference formula (ΔE_{00}) have been identified as 0.8 for PT and 1.8 for AT [30,31].

2.2. Measurement of Light Transmittance Characteristics

Five representative discs (diameter: 4 mm and thickness: 1 mm) from each tested filler-containing resin composite were prepared and immersed in distilled water at 37 °C for 24 h before testing. The two-dimensional distribution of transmitted light intensity for each disc (incidence angle: 0° and measurement range: −90° to +90°) was measured using a goniophotometer (Model GP-200, Murakami Color Research Laboratory, Tokyo, Japan) under controlled conditions (sensitivity: 950 and volume: 508) [32].

2.3. Filler Morphologies of Different Types of Filler Containing Resin Composites

The filler morphology of the four resin composites containing fillers, as well as the ESQ resin composite, was investigated using scanning electron microscopy (SEM; S-4000, Hitachi, Tokyo, Japan). Initially, the resin matrix was dissolved in acetone (Fujifilm Wako Pure Chemicals Industries Co., Ltd., Osaka, Japan). The test specimens were subsequently rinsed with water and allowed to air dry for 5 s. Following additional drying, the specimens were mounted on aluminum stubs and sputter-coated with platinum-palladium (Pt-Pd) ions (E-1030, Hitachi, Tokyo, Japan). Observations were conducted using SEM at an acceleration voltage of 10 kV. The filler morphology was examined at magnifications of ×10,000 and ×20,000.

2.4. Comparison of Two Colorimetric Methods

Instrumental measurements are generally considered to be unreliable between devices [33]. The correlation coefficients were analyzed to evaluate the relationship between the color differences determined by the two measurement approaches: the colorimetric method and the digital photo analysis method. To compare the accuracy of colorimetric measurements (ΔE_{00}) obtained by colorimeter and digital photo analysis methods, statistical analysis was performed using statistical analysis software (SPSS 28.0, IBM, Armonk, NY, USA). The Mann–Whitney U test was performed using the color difference (ΔE_{00}) in the same material and the same shade. The significance level was set at 5%.

2.5. Statistical Analysis

Statistical analysis was performed using statistical software (SPSS 28.0, IBM, Armonk, NY, USA). The significance level was set at 5%. Two-way ANOVA was used to examine the effects of the four materials and four shades on the color difference (ΔE_{00}). If the statistical treatment showed an interaction between the material and shade, a back-test using the Bonferroni method was performed to examine the main effect for each shade.

3. Results

3.1. Evaluation of Shade Matching

Colorimeter results for each material are shown below (Tables 2 and 3). On the white background, L' showed smaller values from A1 to A4, even though the same composite resin was used. C' showed larger values from A1 to A4, H' showed little variation but a slight decreasing trend from A1 to A4, and L' showed a smaller value from A1 to A4, even though the same composite resin was used. On the black background, L' showed small values from A1 to A4, as on the white background, but the values were smaller than on the white background. C' showed an increasing trend, while H' showed a decreasing trend. On both white and black backgrounds, L' showed higher values for EsBF, while C' and H' showed higher values for OCBF in almost all cases.

Table 2. L', C', H', and ΔE_{00} obtained from measurements with the colorimeter (white background).

ESQ's Shade	Code	L'	C'	H'	ΔE_{00}
A1	OCFB	80.2(0.6)	25.5(0.6)	254.0(1.4)	2.10(0.2)
	FiBF	81.0(0.5)	23.6(0.4)	250.7(1.3)	2.09(0.4)
	SDR	81.6(0.8)	20.9(0.6)	247.2(1.9)	3.43(0.5)
	EsBF	82.0(0.4)	22.1(0.4)	250.5(1.5)	2.35(0.5)
A2	OCFB	79.6(0.3)	28.5(0.3)	250.2(1.0)	1.78(0.2)
	FiBF	79.5(0.5)	26.4(0.2)	247.0(1.0)	2.55(0.4)
	SDR	79.6(0.7)	24.0(0.6)	243.8(1.2)	4.02(0.5)
	EsBF	80.5(0.3)	24.5(0.5)	245.0(0.9)	3.28(0.5)
A3	OCFB	76.7(0.4)	30.0(0.3)	248.9(0.7)	0.81(0.4)
	FiBF	76.4(0.6)	28.0(0.5)	245.6(0.9)	3.74(0.4)
	SDR	77.3(0.6)	25.2(0.6)	241.9(1.6)	5.64(0.9)
	EsBF	78.1(0.4)	25.3(0.3)	243.2(1.0)	5.22(0.6)
A4	OCFB	71.6(0.4)	31.4(0.6)	248.6(0.9)	1.74(0.4)
	FiBF	71.0(0.5)	29.4(0.2)	245.1(0.8)	6.90(0.7)
	SDR	72.1(0.6)	27.2(0.6)	242.6(0.9)	7.33(1.5)
	EsBF	72.4(0.5)	26.6(0.6)	241.5(1.1)	6.30(1.6)

Table 3. L', C', H', and ΔE_{00} obtained from measurements with the colorimeter (black background).

ESQ's Shade	Code	L'	C'	H'	ΔE_{00}
A1	OCFB	72.7(0.9)	21.6(0.6)	259.7(2.2)	2.17(0.4)
	FiBF	72.4(0.6)	18.2(0.4)	256.6(2.0)	2.91(0.7)
	SDR	69.6(0.6)	12.4(0.3)	265.5(2.7)	3.99(0.4)
	EsBF	74.0(0.5)	14.2(0.5)	268.2(5.9)	2.79(0.3)
A2	OCFB	68.0(0.5)	20.6(0.3)	260.1(1.6)	1.48(0.5)
	FiBF	66.7(0.4)	17.5(0.1)	258.5(2.4)	3.27(0.3)
	SDR	68.0(0.6)	15.1(0.4)	256.6(3.1)	4.94(0.3)
	EsBF	72.4(0.7)	16.3(0.6)	258.1(3.7)	4.69(0.5)
A3	OCFB	65.9(0.4)	22.6(0.4)	256.7(0.9)	0.64(0.4)
	FiBF	64.7(0.2)	19.6(0.5)	252.0(1.7)	4.87(0.3)
	SDR	66.0(0.5)	16.9(0.4)	250.9(1.6)	6.83(0.6)
	EsBF	70.1(0.8)	17.8(0.8)	252.1(1.8)	5.92(0.7)
A4	OCFB	61.6(0.7)	24.9(0.5)	255.7(0.8)	2.03(0.8)
	FiBF	59.9(0.8)	22.0(0.4)	249.5(0.9)	7.39(0.7)
	SDR	61.4(0.5)	20.0(0.4)	246.3(3.7)	6.43(1.4)
	EsBF	65.2(0.6)	20.1(0.6)	246.9(4.0)	4.97(1.6)

In addition, L', C', H', and color difference (ΔE_{00}) obtained by the digital photo analysis method are shown in Tables 4 and 5.

Table 4. L', C', H', and ΔE_{00} obtained from measurements with the digital photo analysis method (white background).

ESQ's Shade	Code	L'	C'	H'	ΔE_{00}
A1	OCFB	86.6(1.8)	28.6(1.5)	267.2(0.7)	2.65(0.3)
	FiBF	86.9(1.1)	27.3(0.5)	265.3(0.6)	2.20(0.5)
	SDR	87.0(1.0)	24.4(0.6)	265.9(0.3)	2.66(0.4)
	EsBF	86.2(1.6)	24.4(1.0)	265.4(1.4)	2.53(0.21)
A2	OCFB	86.4(1.2)	33.7(0.4)	264.2(0.7)	1.69(0.4)
	FiBF	86.5(0.7)	30.8(0.4)	262.1(0.7)	3.27(0.6)
	SDR	86.9(0.6)	28.8(0.4)	261.9(0.7)	3.20(0.3)
	EsBF	86.6(1.5)	27.8(0.6)	261.5(0.6)	3.94(0.4)

Table 4. *Cont.*

ESQ's Shade	Code	L'	C'	H'	ΔE_{00}
A3	OCFB	83.5(1.2)	35.9(0.4)	261.6(0.6)	0.81(0.3)
	FiBF	83.2(1.7)	32.6(0.5)	258.4(0.7)	4.58(0.4)
	SDR	84.6(0.9)	30.1(0.8)	258.8(0.5)	4.99(0.6)
	EsBF	85.1(0.6)	29.6(0.4)	258.3(0.5)	5.10(0.7)
A4	OCFB	77.2(0.7)	38.4(0.7)	257.0(0.5)	1.73(0.3)
	FiBF	75.7(2.1)	35.1(0.5)	254.2(1.2)	5.35(1.0)
	SDR	77.9(0.7)	32.9(0.6)	254.7(0.5)	5.80(0.7)
	EsBF	77.4(1.5)	31.0(0.7)	253.3(1.1)	5.51(0.9)

Table 5. L', C', H', and ΔE_{00} obtained from measurements with the digital photo analysis method (black background).

ESQ's Shade	Code	L'	C'	H'	ΔE_{00}
A1	OCFB	83.9(0.7)	25.1(0.5)	269.4(0.2)	2.43(0.5)
	FiBF	82.5(1.1)	21.7(0.9)	268.5(0.7)	2.81(0.7)
	SDR	83.8(1.1)	19.5(0.7)	269.2(0.5)	3.27(0.3)
	EsBF	83.8(1.7)	19.7(0.5)	269.4(0.9)	3.72(0.3)
A2	OCFB	81.5(1.1)	28.4(0.9)	266.8(0.7)	1.36(0.4)
	FiBF	81.6(0.9)	24.7(0.7)	266.3(0.7)	3.41(0.4)
	SDR	82.1(1.0)	23.1(0.6)	266.1(0.8)	4.01(0.3)
	EsBF	82.0(2.2)	22.7(0.3)	265.1(1.3)	4.52(0.4)
A3	OCFB	78.5(1.3)	31.1(0.5)	264.2(1.3)	0.78(0.5)
	FiBF	78.2(1.1)	27.8(0.6)	261.2(1.0)	5.54(1.1)
	SDR	79.7(0.7)	24.8(0.5)	262.1(1.3)	5.80(0.8)
	EsBF	79.2(1.6)	24.3(0.5)	261.3(0.7)	5.82(0.6)
A4	OCFB	73.2(1.3)	34.2(0.7)	259.4(1.1)	2.72(0.7)
	FiBF	71.3(1.3)	30.0(0.4)	255.0(1.0)	7.21(1.1)
	SDR	73.0(1.9)	27.5(0.7)	255.9(1.0)	6.99(2.2)
	EsBF	73.5(1.0)	26.8(0.6)	255.0(1.3)	6.33(1.3)

3.2. Color Difference

Furthermore, the color difference (ΔE_{00}) is shown in the graphs in Figures 6 and 7. The color difference (ΔE_{00}) between each material and the ESQ mold is shown below (Figure 6). The color difference (ΔE_{00}) between OCFB and the ESQ mold was 2.10 $\pm$ 0.2 (A1), 1.78 $\pm$ 0.2 (A2), 0.81 $\pm$ 0.4 (A3), and 1.74 $\pm$ 0.4 (A4) for the white background, and 2.17 $\pm$ 0.4 (A1), 1.48 $\pm$ 0.5 (A2), 0.64 $\pm$ 0.4 (A3), and 2.03 $\pm$ 0.8 (A4) for the black background. The ΔE_{00} of OCFB, FiBF, SDR, and EsBF were similar for A1, but the ΔE_{00} of FiBF, SDR, and EsBF became larger as the shade became darker. On the other hand, the ΔE_{00} of OCFB was almost the same as or lower than that of A1, even as the shade became darker. Since the statistical treatment showed an interaction between the material and shade, a Bonferroni back-test for each shade showed that OCFB was significantly lower than FiBF, SDR, and EsBF for A2, A3, and A4 on white and black backgrounds ($p < 0.05$; Figure 6).

The ΔE_{00} of OCFB, FiBF, SDR, and EsBF were similar in the A1 shade, but as the shade became darker, the ΔE_{00} of FiBF, SDR, and EsBF became larger. On the other hand, the ΔE_{00} of OCFB remained almost the same as or lower than that of the A1 shade, even as the shade became darker. Statistical analysis showed an interaction effect between material and shade. When back-testing was performed for each shade using the Bonferroni method, OCFB was significantly lower than FiBF, SDR, and EsBF for shades A2, A3, and A4 on white and black backgrounds ($p < 0.05$; Figure 7).

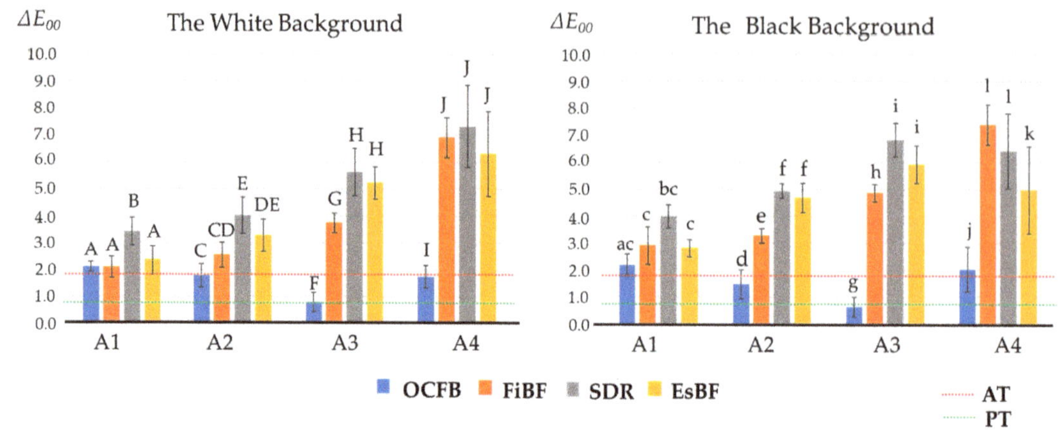

Figure 6. The color difference between four tested materials and resin composites (colorimeter). The perception threshold (PT) in CIEDE2000 was set at 0.8, and the acceptance threshold (AT) at 1.8. The letter differences indicate significant differences between materials of the same shade ($p < 0.05$).

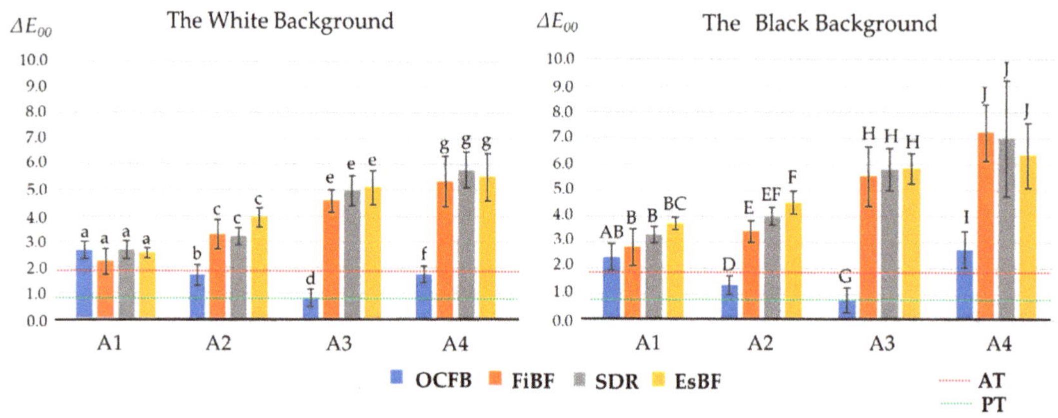

Figure 7. The color difference between the four tested materials and resin composites (digital photo analysis method). The perception threshold (PT) in CIEDE2000 was set at 0.8, and the acceptance threshold (AT) at 1.8. The letter differences indicate significant differences between materials of the same shade ($p < 0.05$).

From the colorimeters, a representative photograph of a sample after each filling is shown below (Figure 8). In the A1 and A2 groups, the filled resin composites generally exhibited a close shade match with the resin mold. Conversely, in the FiBF, SDR, and EsBF groups, an increase in the whiteness of the filled areas became more evident as the shade darkened. In the OCFB group, the filled area demonstrated effective color blending with the surrounding resin, particularly in the A3 and A4 shades. Notably, OCFB consistently achieved superior blending with the surrounding color in these darker shades.

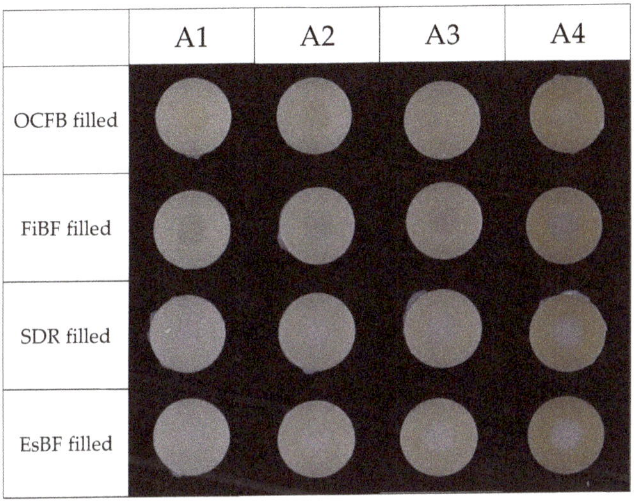

Figure 8. The images of the filled tested resin composites.

3.3. *Measurement of Light Transmittance Characteristics*

The two-dimensional distribution graph of the light transmittance properties of the resin composites tested (Figure 9) revealed that the EsBF-filled group had a wider distribution of light transmission intensity than the other filling groups. This indicates that the diffusion behavior was enhanced compared to the other filling groups. The SDR-filled group also showed a wider distribution of light transmission intensity than the OCFB- and FiBF-filled groups. The horizontal axis of the graph represents the measurement range (°), and the vertical axis represents the intensity (relative value, no unit).

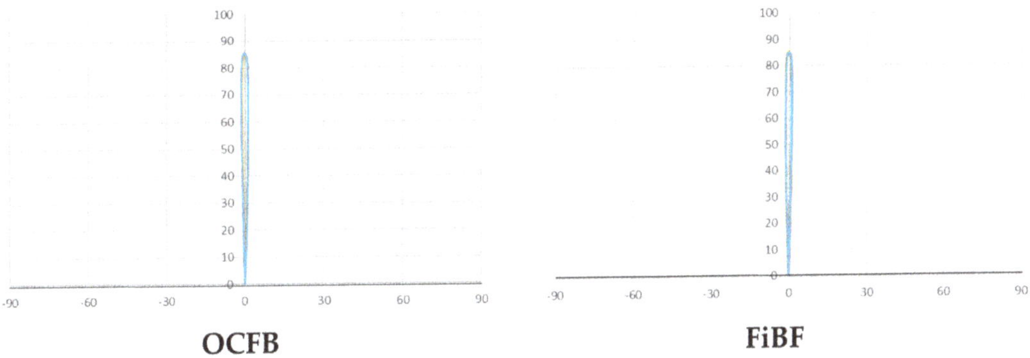

Figure 9. *Cont.*

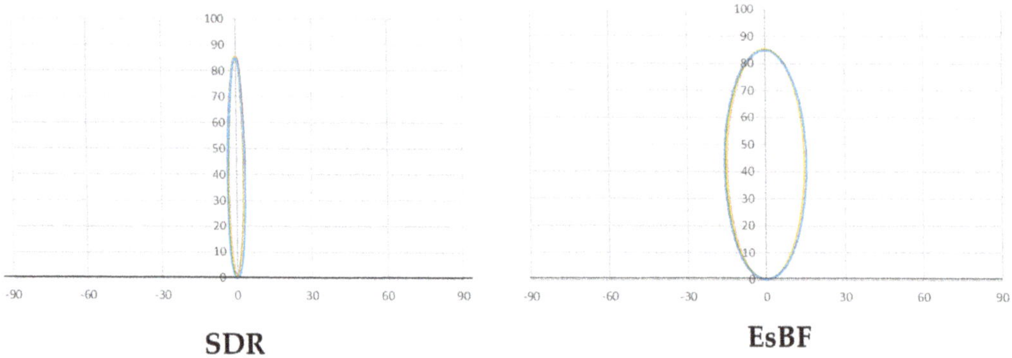

Figure 9. Two-dimensional analysis of light transmittance properties. The horizontal axis of the graph represents the measurement range (°), and the vertical axis represents the intensity (relative value, no unit). The light transmittance of each material was measured five times, with each measurement represented by a distinct line in the graph, differentiated by five colors.

3.4. Filler Morphologies of Different Types of Filler Containing Resin Composites

The SEM images were captured at ×10,000 and ×20,000 magnifications, revealing distinct variations in the morphology, dimensions, and distribution of the filler particles within different resin composites and the resin composite framework (Figure 10).

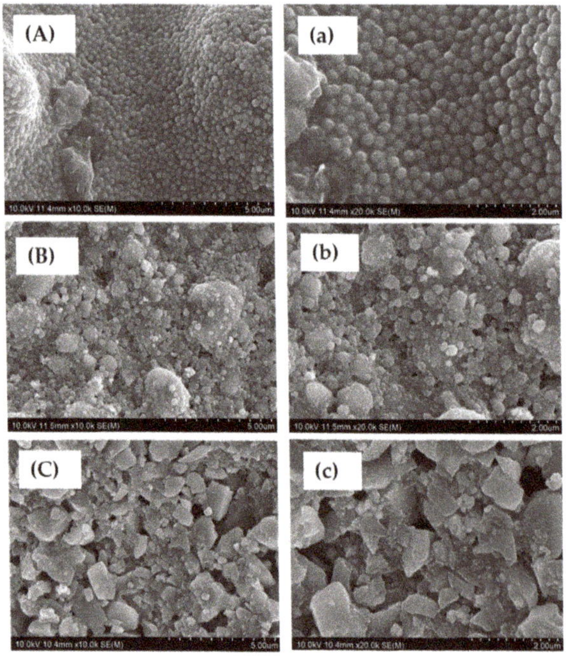

Figure 10. *Cont.*

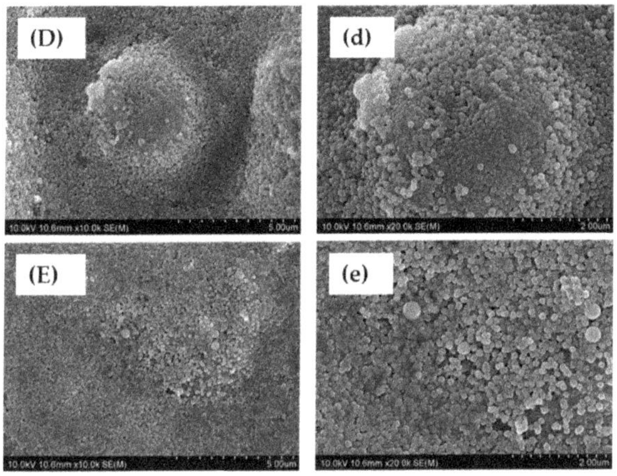

Figure 10. SEM images display the fillers within the tested resin composites and the resin composite frame. The left column presents images at ×10,000 magnification, while the right column showcases images at ×20,000 magnification. (**A**,**a**) OCFB fillers, (**B**,**b**) FiBF fillers, (**C**,**c**) SDR fillers, (**D**,**d**) EsBF fillers, and (**E**,**e**) the ESQ resin composite frame.

OCFB showed a regular distribution of spherical nanofiller particles (Figure 10A,a). FiBF showed aggregates of nanoclusters and nanofillers (Figure 10B,b). SDR showed an irregular distribution of polygonal particles (Figure 10C,c). EsBF showed an image similar to OCFB (Figure 10D,d). ESQ showed spherical nanofiller particles, and occasionally, large irregular spherical particles were observed (Figure 10E,e).

3.5. Comparison of the Two Colorimetric Methods

The correlation coefficients calculated to compare the two methods revealed varying levels of agreement across different conditions. On the white background, the coefficients were as follows: 0.81 for OCFB, 0.80 for FiBF, 0.73 for SDR, and 0.78 for EsBF. These values, ranging from 0.7 to 0.9, indicate a generally strong positive correlation among the tested methods. On the black background, the coefficients were 0.77 for OCFB, 0.85 for FiBF, 0.73 for SDR, and 0.59 for EsBF. While most methods maintained a strong correlation under this condition, EsBF demonstrated a weaker relationship. Overall, the findings suggest that the correlations on the white background were consistently strong, whereas the black background showed greater variability, particularly for EsBF (Table 6).

Table 6. Correlation coefficients of the color differences between colorimeters and digital photo analysis measurement methods.

	OCFB	FiBF	SDR	EsBF
The White Background	0.81	0.80	0.73	0.78
The Black Background	0.77	0.85	0.73	0.59

The values from 0 to less than 0.3 indicate negligible correlation, 0.3 to less than 0.5 indicate a very weak correlation, 0.5 to less than 0.7 indicate a moderate correlation, 0.7 to less than 0.9 indicate a strong correlation, and 0.9 or greater indicate a very strong correlation.

On a white background, no significant differences were observed between the two measurement methods among the nine groups ($p > 0.05$; Figure 11): OCFB (A2, A3, and A4), FiBF (A1), SDR (A3), and EsBF (A1, A3, and A4). However, significant differences were found in the remaining 7 groups ($p < 0.05$). On a black background, no significant differences were found in 11 groups: OCFB (A1, A2, and A3), FiBF (A1, A2, A3, and A4), SDR (A4), and EsBF (A2, A3, and A4; $p > 0.05$; Figure 11). However, significant differences were found in the remaining 5 groups ($p < 0.05$).

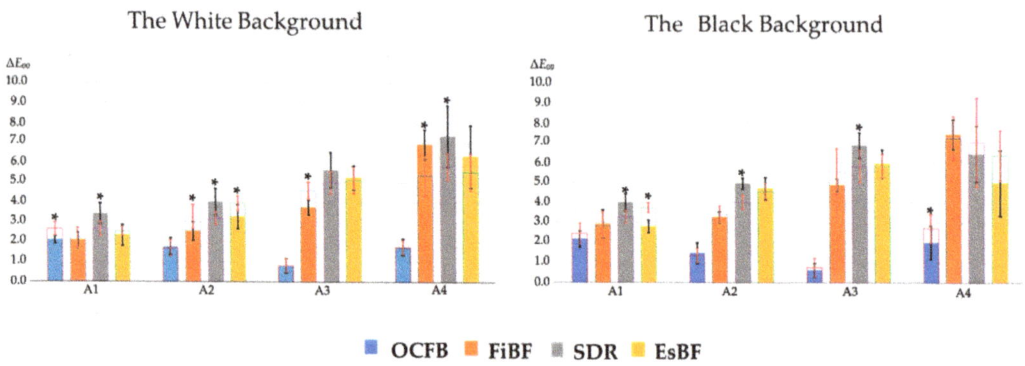

Figure 11. Comparison of colorimeters and CASMATCH (the white and black backgrounds). The solid line in the graph shows the color difference of the colorimeter, and the dashed line shows the color difference of the digital photo analysis method. The black color in the error bar indicates the colorimeter and the red color indicates the digital photo analysis method. * In the figure indicates a significant difference between the two groups ($p < 0.05$).

4. Discussion

In this study, color differences were assessed using two methods: a colorimeter and a digital measurement technique. A comparative analysis revealed a correlation between these two approaches. To enhance both intra- and inter-rater reliability in visual and instrumental tooth color matching, as well as to achieve improved esthetic outcomes, the integration of color-matching instruments as supplementary tools in routine dental practice is recommended [34].

However, specialized instruments, such as colorimeters, are often cost-prohibitive and are not routinely available in most dental clinics [35]. The CASMATCH system, utilizing computerized image-correcting color charts, offers an alternative approach by standardizing the tonality and dimensions of photographic images for the subject. Similarly, Photoshop has demonstrated high validity and reliability for color selection purposes [36].

Given the widespread availability of digital cameras in dental practices [37] and the relatively low cost of CASMATCH compared to colorimeters, the use of CASMATCH in combination with an intraoral camera presents a more accessible and practical alternative for color measurement. This approach may facilitate broader adoption and ease of implementation in clinical settings. In recent years, universal-shade resin composites capable of accommodating a wide range of color shades within a single shade have been introduced to the market. This study focused on evaluating the color compatibility of bulk-fill-type resin composites, which allow for efficient, single-step cavity filling.

Our findings demonstrated that the colorimetric parameters L', C', and H' of the tested resin composites were significantly influenced by the shade of the resin composite mold, particularly as the mold shade darkened. Specifically, L' decreased, C' increased, and H' decreased as the mold shade progressed from A1 to A4. These results align with previous research reporting a decrease in L' values as the cavity depth increased in a simulated fossa cavity of 2 mm in depth. In this study, a deeper simulated first-class cavity of 4 mm was utilized, confirming a consistent trend of diminished lightness with increasing cavity depth [21].

The observed changes in color parameters can be attributed to intrinsic properties of the resin composites, such as light scattering, absorption, reflectance, and translucency. When light interacts with a resin composite, it encounters the resin matrix, filler particles, pigments, and background color, which collectively influence the perceived color [38]. Notably, the interplay of light scattering and absorption modifies the background color through a filtering effect governed by the translucency of the material [23]. Furthermore, the thickness of the resin composite and the reflectance of the underlying background were critical in determining the resultant color coordinates [23]. These principles also apply to universal-shade resins, as demonstrated in our study.

Additionally, scanning electron microscopy (SEM) analysis revealed variations in filler morphology among the examined materials. For instance, OCFB and EsBF exhibited fillers with similar shapes but differing sizes. The refractive index of the filler and matrix, as well as the light diffusivity of the resin composite, are influenced by the filler content and matrix composition. The optical diffusivity of EsBF was notably higher than that of the other tested materials, including OCFB. This difference may be attributed to variations in the filler particle size and distribution.

Previous research has indicated that resin composites with smaller, irregularly shaped fillers generally exhibit higher light transmittance and sharper angular distribution peaks compared to those with larger, spherical fillers. Interestingly, while SDR contains irregular fillers, its diffusivity was surpassed by EsBF in this study. This discrepancy is likely due to the particle size of the fillers in EsBF, emphasizing the importance of filler morphology in determining optical properties.

In conclusion, the interaction of material properties, such as filler shape, size, and distribution, with optical characteristics underscores the complexity of color compatibility in resin composites. These findings provide valuable insights into the factors influencing the performance of universal-shade and bulk-fill resins in restorative dentistry.

While the CIELAB formula (ΔE_{ab}) is frequently applied in dental procedures due to its established reliability in quantifying color, the CIEDE2000 formula (ΔE_{00}) offers a more advanced approach [23,26]. The latter provides a closer correlation with perceptual color differences, as judged by human vision [23,25,39]. Therefore, the CIEDE2000 formula was selected for use in this study to assess color differences, considering its demonstrated advantages in aligning with human visual perception.

As mentioned earlier, corresponding values in the CIEDE2000 color difference formula (ΔE_{00}) have been identified as 0.8 for PT and 1.8 for AT [30,31]. The color difference measurements of OCFB, as evaluated using a colorimeter, demonstrated satisfactory color matching, with ΔE_{00} values below the acceptable threshold (AT) for shades A2 and A4 against a white background and for shade A2 against a black background. Additionally, OCFB exhibited the best color matching, with ΔE_{00} values below the perceptibility threshold (PT) for shade A3 on both white and black backgrounds. Similarly, the CASMATCH analysis indicated that OCFB achieved good color differences below the AT for shades A2, A3, and A4 on the white background, as well as for shade A2 on the black background. Notably, the best color difference, below the PT, was observed for shade A3 on the black background.

In the A1 shade measured with a colorimeter, the ΔE_{00} values of OCFB, FiBF, and EsBF were nearly identical when measured against the black background, while SDR exhibited significantly higher values ($p < 0.05$). On the white background, OCFB showed significantly lower color differences compared to SDR ($p < 0.05$).

Omnichroma Flow contains uniform spherical ultra-nanofiller particles with an average diameter of 260 nanometers and, furthermore, contains no pigment and has high transparency [40].

Similar to Omnichroma and Omnichroma Flow, OCFB also contains uniform spherical ultra-nanofiller particles with an average diameter of 260 nanometers and contains no pigments. Furthermore, the bulk-fill-type resin composite allows filling of 4 mm cavities in a batch.

The structural color depends on the distribution of refractive indices, and the difference between the matrix and filler refractive indices must be considered, with the refractive index of the filler particles ranging from 1.47 to 1.52, corresponding to the refractive index of the resin matrix [10]. Arai et al. also found that the appearance of the structural color depends not only on the size of the filler but also on the filler content [41]: the filler content of Omnichroma Flow is 70% and the matrix resin is UDMA [40]. In our previous study, Omnichroma Flow showed a better color match compared to other esthetic resin composites at a cavity depth of 2 mm [20]. This was due to the structural coloration. On the other hand, the filler content of OCFB was 69%, which is almost the same as that of Omnichroma Flow, and the matrix resins are UDMA and TEGDMA. This indicates that OCFB also has a characteristic structural color, which may serve as an explanation for the better esthetic results observed in this study. In other words, OCFB contains spherical ultra-nanofiller particles with an average diameter of 260 nm, which contribute to red–yellow wavelength reflection and contribute to shade matching.

A previous study showed that shade matching of resin composites is facilitated by the light transmittance and light diffusivity of the material [42].

The color of a resin composite is affected by the light scattering, absorption properties, reflectance, and translucency of the material [43]. When light enters a resin composite, it interacts with the resin matrix, fillers, pigments, and background color and is simultaneously perceived as a specific color [38]. The interaction of light scattering and absorption changes the color parameters due to the filtering effect caused by the translucency of the material, affecting the background color [34]. Both the thickness of the resin composite and the reflectance of the background play an important role in determining the color coordinates [23].

A previous study reported a statistically significant difference ($p < 0.05$) in translucency between resin composites with and without pigments, with translucency decreasing as the pigment concentration increased [44]. There is also a negative correlation between material thickness and transparency, with transparency decreasing with increasing thickness [44]. This is because as material thickness increases, light travels a longer path through the sample and encounters more interfaces between particles and the matrix, resulting in increased scattering at these interfaces [45].

Nevertheless, in bulk-filled resin composites, a thickness of 4 mm can be polymerized directly according to the manufacturer. This may be explained by its satisfactory translucency (OCFB, FiBF, and SDR) [45]. The compatibility of the refractive index of the resin matrix and filler particles is important to achieve high translucency in resin composites [46]. Therefore, future studies will need to evaluate the light transmittance and spectral reflectance of each bulk-filled resin composite using a spectrophotometer.

In our previous study, the flowable type of esthetic resin composite, Omnichroma Flow, showed superior color matching compared to other esthetic resin composites at a cavity depth of 2 mm [20]. On the other hand, a cavity depth of 4 mm was used in this study. The results showed that the bulk-filled resin composite OCFB-001 exhibited perceptible color matching up to the A1–A4 shades at a cavity depth of 4 mm, while other flowable resin composites exhibited perceptible color matching at the A1 shade, but for the surrounding cavity shades A2, A3, and A4, the color differences were discernible.

This may be because OCFB does not contain pigments and exhibits excellent color matching due to its coloration by structural color, while the other three materials have adjusted the amounts of pigments and the refractive index of the matrix and filler to match a white shade, such as A1.

Depending on its structural color, OCFB reflects yellow wavelengths in light-color cavities, such as the A1 shade, and red wavelengths in dark-color cavities, such as the A4 shade, in harmony with the cavity wall color.

The other three materials, on the other hand, would have had perceptible color matching in the lighter materials, such as the A1 shade, but the pigments and low lightness would have made harmonization more difficult and the color differences more pronounced.

Nevertheless, this study examined the color matching of only universal shades and did not compare the results with the results of actual dentists' rigorous shade matching and filling. For the three commercial materials used, it is possible that they may have shades that may better match certain colors. Conventional composite resin restorations for a cavity depth of 4 mm are more difficult to restore because light penetration into the cavity floor is weak and prone to under-polymerization. In addition, deeper cavities are usually darker in color than the cavity floor, and the use of the cavity floor for light reflection to improve esthetics also has an effect, making color matching difficult [46]. As mentioned earlier, OCFB was shown to have good tonal conformity in a 4 mm simulated cavity. From this, it can be inferred that satisfactory translucency was achieved. In this study, a 4 mm monochromatic simulated Class I cavity was used, but this is not the case in Class II–IV cavities, which do not have a dentin backing. Further study is needed because in natural teeth, the color varies among the superficial enamel, the dentin behind it, and the dentin adjacent to the pulp.

Based on the above, the null hypothesis that "there is no significant difference in color match and color parameters among the tested universal-shade flowable bulk-fill composite resins in the 4 mm standard cavity" was rejected.

The application of filler forms for shade matching represents a recent advancement in dental material science. This technique relies on the light absorption and emission properties of resin composites to achieve precise shade matching. Notably, super nano-filled resin composites, which derive their shading primarily from the structural color, present a potential advantage due to the alignment of their filler particles with visible-light wavelengths. This alignment minimizes photochemical degradation and reduces color distortion over time, thereby enhancing shade stability [20]. Consequently, the incorporation of optically controlled filler-based systems (OCFBs) may streamline treatment by reducing the time required for shade-matching and layering techniques. Furthermore, this approach may lower the technical sensitivity of the process, enabling practitioners of varying skill levels to achieve optimal aesthetic outcomes with greater ease. However, as this investigation was conducted under in vitro conditions, further research in clinical settings is imperative to validate these findings and assess their practical implications.

5. Conclusions

OCFB-001 demonstrated excellent color compatibility within the shade range of A2 to A4, and comparable color compatibility to existing universal bulk-fill resin composites in the A1 shade. Additionally, the use of OCFB-001 is expected to streamline procedures and enhance esthetic outcomes. These findings underscore its clinical utility and suggest potential future research directions, such as validation under natural lighting or using natural teeth as testing conditions.

Author Contributions: Conceptualization, H.K. and C.K.; methodology, C.K. and R.Y.; software, R.Y. and D.W.; validation, D.W., Y.Y. and A.T.; formal analysis, Y.T., F.C. and M.Y.; investigation, H.K., Y.T., R.Y., D.W., Y.Y. and F.C.; resources, C.K. and H.S.; data curation, H.K. and C.K.; writing—original draft preparation, H.K., C.K., Y.T. and R.Y.; writing—review and editing, H.K., C.K., Y.T. and R.Y.; visualization, H.K. and R.Y.; supervision, M.Y. and H.S.; project administration, C.K. and A.T.; funding acquisition, C.K. and H.S. All authors have read and agreed to the published version of the manuscript.

Funding: This study was supported in part by Grants-in-Aid for Regional R&D Proposal-Based Program from Northern Advancement Center for Science & Technology of Hokkaido Japan.

Institutional Review Board Statement: Not applicable.

Informed Consent Statement: Not applicable.

Data Availability Statement: The original contributions presented in the study are included in the article, further inquiries can be directed to the corresponding author.

Conflicts of Interest: The authors declare no conflicts of interest.

References

1. Sidhu, S.K.; Ikeda, T.; Omata, Y.; Fujita, M.; Sano, H. Change of color and translucency by light curing in resin composites. *Oper. Dent.* **2006**, *31*, 598–603. [CrossRef] [PubMed]
2. Lucchese, A.; Storti, E. Morphological characteristics of primary enamel surfaces versus permanent enamel surfaces: SEM digital analysis. *Eur. J. Paediatr. Dent.* **2011**, *12*, 179–183. [PubMed]

3. Ikeda, T.; Sidhu, S.K.; Omata, Y.; Fujita, M.; Sano, H. Colour and translucency of opaque-shades and body-shades of resin composites. *Eur. J. Oral Sci.* **2005**, *113*, 170–173. [CrossRef] [PubMed]
4. Miotti, L.L.; Santos, I.S.; Nicoloso, G.F.; Pozzobon, R.T.; Susin, A.H.; Durand, L.B. The Use of Resin Composite Layering Technique to Mask Discolored Background: A CIELAB/CIEDE2000 Analysis. *Oper. Dent.* **2017**, *42*, 165–174. [CrossRef] [PubMed]
5. Perez, B.G.; Gaidarji, B.; Palm, B.G.; Ruiz-López, J.; Pérez, M.M.; Durand, L.B. Masking ability of resin composites: Effect of the layering strategy and substrate color. *J. Esthet. Restor. Dent.* **2022**, *34*, 1206–1212. [CrossRef] [PubMed]
6. Hardan, L.; Bourgi, R.; Cuevas-Suárez, C.E.; Lukomska-Szymanska, M.; Monjarás-Ávila, A.J.; Zarow, M.; Jakubowicz, N.; Jorquera, G.; Ashi, T.; Mancino, D.; et al. Novel Trends in Dental Color Match Using Different Shade Selection Methods: A Systematic Review and Meta-Analysis. *Materials* **2022**, *15*, 468. [CrossRef] [PubMed] [PubMed Central]
7. Abdelraouf, R.M.; Habib, N.A. Color matching and blending effect of universal shade bulk fill resin composite in resin composite models and natural teeth. *BioMed Res. Int.* **2016**, *2016*, 4183432. [CrossRef]
8. Lee, Y.K. Influence of scattering/absorption characteristics on the color of resin composites. *Dent. Mater.* **2007**, *23*, 124–131. [CrossRef]
9. Lee, Y.K.; Lu, H.; Powers, J.M. Measurement of opalescent property of resin composites. *Dent. Mater.* **2005**, *21*, 1068–1074. [CrossRef]
10. Oivanen, M.; Keulemans, F.; Garoushi, S.; Vallittu, P.K.; Lassila, L. The effect of refractive index of fillers and polymer matrix on translucency and color matching of dental resin composite. *Biomater. Investig. Dent.* **2021**, *8*, 48–53. [CrossRef] [PubMed] [PubMed Central]
11. Sakaguchi, R.L.; Douglas, W.H.; Peters, M.C. Curing light performance and polymerization of composite restorative materials. *J. Dent.* **1992**, *20*, 183–188. [CrossRef] [PubMed]
12. Pilo, R.; Oelgiesser, D.; Cardash, H.S. A survey of output intensity and potential for depth of cure among light-curing units in clinical use. *J. Dent.* **1999**, *27*, 235–241. [CrossRef] [PubMed]
13. Flury, S.; Peutzfeldt, A.; Lussi, A. Influence of increment thickness on microhardness and dentin bond strength of bulk fill resin composites. *Dent. Mater.* **2014**, *30*, 1104–1112. [CrossRef] [PubMed]
14. Lucena, C.; Ruiz-López, J.; Pulgar, R.; Della Bona, A.; Pérez, M.M. Optical behavior of one-shaded resin-based composites. *Dent. Mater.* **2021**, *37*, 840–848. [CrossRef] [PubMed]
15. Lowe, R.A. OMNICHROMA: One Composite That Covers All Shades for an Anterior Tooth. *Compend. Contin. Educ. Dent.* **2019**, *40* (Suppl. S1), 8–10. [PubMed]
16. Graf, N.; Ilie, N. Long-term mechanical stability and light transmission characteristics of one shade resin-based composites. *J. Dent.* **2022**, *116*, 103915. [CrossRef] [PubMed]
17. Pereira Sanchez, N.; Powers, J.M.; Paravina, R.D. Instrumental and visual evaluation of the color adjustment potential of resin composites. *J. Esthet. Restor. Dent.* **2019**, *31*, 465–470. [CrossRef] [PubMed]
18. Altınışık, H.; Özyurt, E. Instrumental and visual evaluation of the color adjustment potential of different single-shade resin composites to human teeth of various shades. *Clin. Oral Investig.* **2023**, *27*, 889–896. [CrossRef] [PubMed]
19. Chen, F.; Toida, Y.; Islam, R.; Alam, A.; Chowdhury, A.F.M.A.; Yamauti, M.; Sano, H. Evaluation of shade matching of a novel supra-nano filled esthetic resin composite employing structural color using simplified simulated clinical cavities. *J. Esthet. Restor. Dent.* **2021**, *33*, 874–883. [CrossRef]
20. Chen, F.; Wu, D.; Islam, R.; Toida, Y.; Kawamoto, C.; Yamauti, M.; Sano, H. Evaluation of Color and Spectral Behavior of a Novel Flowable Resin Composite after Water Aging: An In Vitro Study. *Materials* **2022**, *15*, 4102. [CrossRef] [PubMed] [PubMed Central]
21. Kang, S.; Ryu, S.Y.; Kim, K.M.; Park, S.H. Effect of thickness on the translucency of resin-based composites and glass-ceramics. *Dent. Mater. J.* **2023**, *42*, 30–41. [CrossRef] [PubMed]
22. Tsubone, M.; Nakajima, M.; Hosaka, K.; Foxton, R.M.; Tagami, J. Color shifting at the border of resin composite restorations in human tooth cavity. *Dent. Mater.* **2012**, *28*, 811–817. [CrossRef] [PubMed]
23. Medeiros, J.A.; Pecho, O.E.; Pérez, M.M.; Carrillo-Pérez, F.; Herrera, L.J.; Della Bona, A. Influence of background color on color perception in dentistry. *J. Dent.* **2021**, *108*, 103640. [CrossRef] [PubMed]
24. Witt, K. Excel Spreadsheet Implementation of the CIEDE2000 Color Difference Formula (Including Test Data). Available online: http://www.rit.edu/cos/colorscience/rc_usefuldata.php (accessed on 19 August 2024).
25. Del Mar Perez, M.; Ghinea, R.; Herrera, L.J.; Ionescu, A.M.; Pomares, H.; Pulgar, R.; Paravina, R.D. Dental ceramics: A CIEDE2000 acceptability thresholds for lightness, chroma, and hue differences. *J. Dent.* **2011**, *39* (Suppl. S3), e37–e44. [CrossRef] [PubMed]
26. Gómez-Polo, C.; Portillo Muñoz, M.; Lorenzo Luengo, M.C.; Vicente, P.; Galindo, P.; Martín Casado, A.M. Comparison of the CIELab and CIEDE2000 color difference formulas. *J. Prosthet. Dent.* **2016**, *115*, 65–70. [CrossRef] [PubMed]
27. Paravina, R.D.; Ghinea, R.; Herrera, L.J.; Bona, A.D.; Igiel, C.; Linninger, M.; Sakai, M.; Takahashi, H.; Tashkandi, E.; Perez Mdel, M. Color difference thresholds in dentistry. *J. Esthet. Restor. Dent.* **2015**, *27* (Suppl. S1), S1–S9. [CrossRef] [PubMed]
28. Paravina, R.D.; Pérez, M.M.; Ghinea, R. Acceptability and perceptibility thresholds in dentistry: A comprehensive review of clinical and research applications. *J. Esthet. Restor. Dent.* **2019**, *31*, 103–112. [CrossRef] [PubMed]
29. Khashayar, G.; Bain, P.A.; Salari, S.; Dozic, A.; Kleverlaan, C.J.; Feilzer, A.J. Perceptibility and acceptability thresholds for color differences in dentistry. *J. Dent.* **2014**, *42*, 637–644. [CrossRef] [PubMed]
30. Xu, B.T.; Zhang, B.; Kang, Y.; Wang, Y.N.; Li, Q. Applicability of CIELAB/CIEDE2000 formula in visual color assessments of metal-ceramic restorations. *J. Dent.* **2012**, *40* (Suppl. S1), e3–e9. [CrossRef] [PubMed]

31. Paravina, R.D.; Majkic, G.; Imai, F.H.; Powers, J.M. Optimization of tooth color and shade guide design. *J. Prosthodont.* **2007**, *16*, 269–276. [CrossRef] [PubMed]
32. Horie, K.; Nakajima, M.; Hosaka, K.; Kainose, K.; Tanaka, A.; Foxton, R.M.; Tagami, J. Influences of composite-composite join on light transmission characteristics of layered resin composites. *Dent. Mater.* **2012**, *28*, 204–211. [CrossRef] [PubMed]
33. Sarafianou, A.; Kamposiora, P.; Papavasiliou, G.; Goula, H. Matching repeatability and interdevice agreement of 2 intraoral spectrophotometers. *J. Prosthet. Dent.* **2012**, *107*, 178–185. [CrossRef] [PubMed]
34. Igiel, C.; Lehmann, K.M.; Ghinea, R.; Weyhrauch, M.; Hangx, Y.; Scheller, H.; Paravina, R.D. Reliability of visual and instrumental color matching. *J. Esthet. Restor. Dent.* **2017**, *29*, 303–308. [CrossRef] [PubMed]
35. Sampaio, C.S.; Atria, P.J.; Hirata, R.; Jorquera, G. Variability of color matching with different digital photography techniques and a gray reference card. *J. Prosthet. Dent.* **2019**, *121*, 333–339. [CrossRef] [PubMed]
36. Mohammadi, A.; Bakhtiari, Z.; Mighani, F.; Bakhtiari, F. Validity and reliability of tooth color selection by smartphone photography and software applications. *J. Indian Prosthodont. Soc.* **2021**, *21*, 281–286. [CrossRef] [PubMed] [PubMed Central]
37. Chu, S.J.; Trushkowsky, R.D.; Paravina, R.D. Dental color matching instruments and systems. Review of clinical and research aspects. *J. Dent.* **2010**, *38* (Suppl. S2), e2–e16. [CrossRef] [PubMed]
38. Arimoto, A.; Nakajima, M.; Hosaka, K.; Nishimura, K.; Ikeda, M.; Foxton, R.M.; Tagami, J. Translucency, opalescence and light transmission characteristics of light-cured resin composites. *Dent. Mater.* **2010**, *26*, 1090–1097. [CrossRef] [PubMed]
39. Ghinea, R.; Pérez, M.M.; Herrera, L.J.; Rivas, M.J.; Yebra, A.; Paravina, R.D. Color difference thresholds in dental ceramics. *J. Dent.* **2010**, *38* (Suppl. S2), e57–e64. [CrossRef] [PubMed]
40. Technical Report—OMNICHROMA FLOW. Available online: https://omnichromaflow.com/wp-content/uploads/2021/02/OMNICHROMA-FLOW-Tech-Report.pdf (accessed on 2 October 2024).
41. Arai, Y.; Kurokawa, H.; Takamizawa, T.; Tsujimoto, A.; Saegusa, M.; Yokoyama, M.; Miyazaki, M. Evaluation of structural coloration of experimental flowable resin composites. *J. Esthet. Restor. Dent.* **2021**, *33*, 284–293. [CrossRef] [PubMed]
42. Aida, A.; Nakajima, M.; Seki, N.; Kano, Y.; Foxton, R.M.; Tagami, J. Effect of enamel margin configuration on color change of resin composite restoration. *Dent. Mater. J.* **2016**, *35*, 675–683. [CrossRef] [PubMed]
43. Leyva Del Rio, D.; Johnston, W.M. Optical characteristics of experimental dental composite resin materials. *J. Dent.* **2022**, *118*, 103949. [CrossRef] [PubMed]
44. Azhar, G.; Haas, K.; Wood, D.J.; van Noort, R.; Moharamzadeh, K. The Effects of Colored Pigments on the Translucency of Experimental Dental Resin Composites. *Eur. J. Prosthodont. Restor. Dent.* **2019**, *27*, 3–9. [CrossRef] [PubMed]
45. Nakajima, M.; Arimoto, A.; Prasansuttiporn, T.; Thanatvarakorn, O.; Foxton, R.M.; Tagami, J. Light transmission characteristics of dentine and resin composites with different thickness. *J. Dent.* **2012**, *40* (Suppl. S2), e77–e82. [CrossRef] [PubMed]
46. Son, S.A.; Park, J.K.; Seo, D.G.; Ko, C.C.; Kwon, Y.H. How do light attenuation and filler content affect the microhardness polymerization shrinkage and translucency of bulk-fill composites? *Clin. Oral Investig.* **2017**, *21*, 559–565. [CrossRef] [PubMed]

materials

Article

The Effect of Inorganic Filler Content on the Properties of BPA-Free Bulk-Fill Dental Resin Composites

Huilin Deng, Fang Liu and Jingwei He *

School of Materials Science and Engineering, South China University of Technology, Guangzhou 510641, China; 202320118059@mail.scut.edu.cn (H.D.); mcfliu@126.com (F.L.)
* Correspondence: msjwhe@scut.edu.cn

Abstract: This study aimed to enhance the performance of dental resin composites (DRCs) by increasing the content of inorganic fillers while addressing potential health risks associated with Bisphenol A (BPA). To achieve this, the BPA-based resin monomer Bis-GMA was replaced with BPA-free Bis-EFMA. The study then explored the impact of varying inorganic filler contents on the physiochemical properties of Bis-EFMA-based bulk-fill dental resin composites (BF-DRCs). Four distinct Bis-EFMA-based BF-DRCs were formulated, each with different inorganic filler contents ranging from 70 wt% to 76 wt%. The study tested the depth of cure (DOC), double-bond conversion (DC), water sorption (WS), solubility (SL), and cytotoxicity of the system. It notably investigated the effects of increasing filler content on mechanical properties through flexural strength (FS), flexural modulus (FM), Vickers microhardness (VHN), and wear resistance, as well as the impact on polymerization shrinkage, including volumetric shrinkage (VS) and shrinkage stress (SS). To assess the commercial application potential of Bis-EFMA-based BF-DRC, the research used the commercially available BF-DRC Filtek Bulk-Fill Posterior (FBF) as a control. The results indicated that a higher filler content did not affect the DOC of Bis-EFMA-based BF-DRCs. Inorganic fillers at higher concentrations significantly enhanced overall mechanical properties while significantly reducing volumetric shrinkage (VS; $p < 0.05$). When the concentration of inorganic fillers in the resin system reached 76 wt%, most of the performance of the Bis-EFMA-based BF-DRC surpassed that of the commercial control FBF, except for FS, FM, and SS. These findings highlight the potential of Bis-EFMA-based BF-DRC as a long-term restorative material for dental applications.

Keywords: bulk-fill resin composites; inorganic filler content; physicochemical properties

1. Introduction

Resin-based materials have gained significant traction in various dental applications. They are most commonly used in dental prosthetics, where dental resin composites (DRCs) that match tooth color adhere to dental tissue using adhesives. This advancement has led to DRCs replacing amalgam fillings as the preferred solution for repairing wear, trauma, or caries [1]. DRCs consist of two main components, including resin matrix (containing monomer, photopolymerization initiators, promoter, inhibitor, and colorant) and inorganic filler particles, which provide most of the DRCs' mechanical properties and the desired optical and radiopaque properties required [2]. Common monomers in DRCs consist mainly of a mixture of monomers, including Bisphenol A glycidyl methacrylate (Bis-GMA), urethane dimethacrylate (UDMA), and triethyleneglycol dimethacrylate (TEGDMA).

Despite their successful application in dental practices for several decades, concerns regarding the safety and biocompatibility of dental resin composites (DRCs) persist. These concerns are primarily attributed to the release of incompletely polymerized and unpolymerized compounds, including residual monomers, which have the potential to diffuse through dentinal tubules, be absorbed into the pulp, or be released into the oral cavity and subsequently ingested [3]. Furthermore, the release of Bisphenol A (BPA), an endocrine disruptor, and the associated health risks have garnered significant attention [4–6]. Numerous studies have indicated that BPA, a degradation product present in most dental resin composites, can lead to severe health issues, such as fetal growth restriction [7], anxiety and depression [8], obesity [9], and adverse immune effects [10]. Bis-GMA, a BPA derivative, is widely used in DRCs due to its favorable mechanical properties post-polymerization, low volumetric shrinkage, low volatility, and high refractive index [11]. However, removing this monomer from resin formulations and reducing resin content may help mitigate the health risks associated with BPA [12]. Although UDMA, a non-BPA derivative monomer, can partially or fully substitute Bis-GMA, UDMA-based dental resin composite exhibit higher volumetric shrinkage compared to those containing Bis-GMA [13]. Therefore, further research is necessary to explore alternative monomers to Bis-GMA that can provide similar or improved properties without the associated health risks [14–17].

He and his colleagues developed a BPA-free high-refractive-index resin monomer, called Bis-EFMA [18]. This innovative monomer boasts a molecular weight and rigid phenyl structure that contribute to enhanced mechanical properties. Its high refractive index aligns well with fillers, improving light transmission in DRCs. Bis-EFMA serves not only as an excellent alternative to Bis-GMA but also as a resin monomer for producing bulk-fill dental resin composites (BF-DRCs), which are designed for placement in increments of 4 or 5 mm, enabling efficient one-step curing [19]. BF-DRCs can overcome time-consuming incremental placement techniques, offering low polymerization stress and outstanding physical properties, excelling in wear resistance, functionality, and aesthetics [20]. Numerous studies have validated the effective performance of the Bis-EFMA resin monomer. Hatipoğlu et al. investigated the elution, microhardness, and roughness of Bis-EFMA-based DRCs, concluding that Bis-EFMA serves as a viable alternative to Bis-GMA in commercial DRCs due to its superior color stability [21], reduced monomer elution, and increased microhardness [22]. Zhang et al. formulated resin systems utilizing Bis-EFMA and TEGDMA in varying proportions, which demonstrated superior refractive indices over Bis-GMA-based systems, alongside improved flexural modulus and minimized volumetric shrinkage and shrinkage stress, enabling functionality as BF-DRCs [23]. Ma et al. examined various properties of DRCs incorporating Bis-EFMA by mixing five distinct ratios of UDMA, revealing that the depth of cure of these composites meets the requirements for BF-DRCs with suitable resin formulations. Furthermore, specific ratios of Bis-EFMA/UDMA-based DRCs offer benefits, such as enhanced flexural modulus and flow, decreased polymerization shrinkage, exceptional biocompatibility, and favorable adhesive properties, compared to Bis-GMA-based DRCs [24]. In clinical assessments, the incorporation of Bis-EFMA demonstrated remarkable biocompatibility and color stability. It provided edge-sealing performance comparable to the clinically utilized BF-DRCs, along with commendable mechanical strength and wear resistance [25]. With these impressive attributes, Bis-EFMA is poised for application in commercial DRCs, particularly those designated for use as BF-DRCs.

Safe and efficient resin composites are among the research objectives in dental materials. Building upon the foundational work conducted on Bis-EFMA, this study set its sights on propelling the commercial application of Bis-EFMA-based DRCs by augmenting their mechanical properties and biocompatibility. The study delves into the ramifications of augmenting the inorganic filler content within Bis-EFMA-based DRCs. This extensive research explores crucial parameters for evaluating the performance of resin composite. It examines aspects such as the depth of cure (DOC), double-bond conversion (DC), water sorption (WS), solubility (SL), and cytotoxicity. The study primarily focuses on how augmenting the content of inorganic fillers influences the mechanical properties of BF-DRCs. It includes features such as flexural strength (FS), flexural modulus (FM), Vickers microhardness (VHN), and wear resistance, along with the effects on polymerization shrinkage. To test the validity of our assumptions, we formulated three null hypotheses: (1) Elevating the inorganic filler content would alter the bulk filling performance of Bis-EFMA-based DRCs, (2) augmenting the inorganic filler content would not exert a significant influence on the mechanical properties of Bis-EFMA-based DRCs, and (3) enhancing the inorganic filler content would not notably affect the polymerization shrinkage of Bis-EFMA-based DRCs. Through rigorous experimentation and analysis, this study aims to uncover the optimal balance of inorganic filler content that would propel Bis-EFMA-based BF-DRCs to the forefront of dental material innovation, combining good operability, exceptional mechanical strength, and minimal polymerization shrinkage.

2. Materials and Methods

2.1. Materials

The 9,9-Bis[4-((2-(2-methacryloyloxy)ethyl-carbamate)ethoxy)phenyl] fluorene (Bis-EFMA) was prepared by the method provided in the literature [18] (Figure 1). Triethyleneglycol dimethacrylate (TEGDMA) and urethane dimethacrylate (UDMA) were sourced from the Tokyo Chemical Industry, Tokyo, Japan. Camphor quinone (CQ) was acquired from J&K Scientific, Beijing, China. N, N′-dimethylaminoethyl methacrylate (DMAEMA) was procured from J&K Scientific, Beijing, China. Silanated inorganic glass fillers (SCHOTT® UltraFine, GM 27884, with 6% silane, a particle size of 0.7 μm, and a refractive index of 1.53) were obtained from SCHOTT AG in Mainz, Germany. As a reference material, 3 M™ Filtek™ Bulk-Fill Posterior (FBF) was purchased from 3 M Espe in St. Paul, MN, USA. The curing light used was the CL 2500, which operates in a wavelength range of 400–520 nm and at an intensity of approximately 550 mW cm^{-2}, manufactured by 3 M Co., MN, USA.

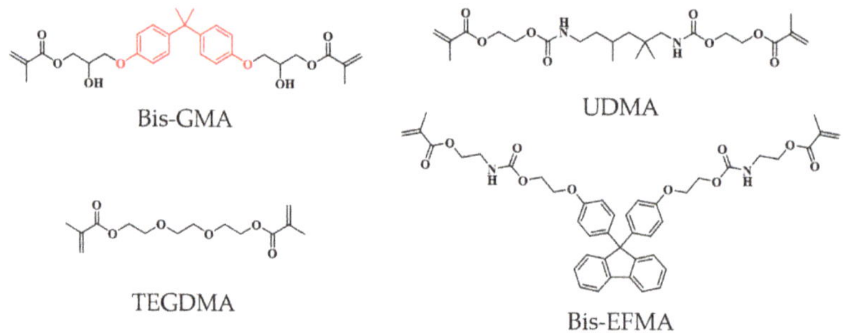

Figure 1. The structures of the resin monomer [13,18]. In the structural formula of Bis-GMA, the red-highlighted section represents the core structure of Bisphenol A. The chemical formulas were drawn using ChemDraw 18.0.

2.2. *Preparation of Dental Resin Matrix and Composites*

The dental resin systems without fillers were formulated based on the proportions detailed in Table 1. Each component was carefully weighed and thoroughly mixed using a magnetic stirrer. The resin matrix composition was determined with reference to prior research [23,24], consisting of UDMA, Bis-EFMA, and TEGDMA in weight percentages of 36 wt%, 24 wt%, and 40 wt%, respectively. To prepare the DRCs, silanated inorganic glass fillers were blended with the resin matrix using a high-speed mixer (ZHI DI TECH, Shenzhen, China) at 2800 rpm until a homogeneous mixture was achieved (Figure 2). For comparison, FBF was selected as the commercial control material, which features a matrix composed of Bis-GMA, UDMA, Bisphenol A ethoxylate dimethacrylate (Bis-EMA), TEGDMA, and EDMAB (RI: 1.52), and filler content of silica, zirconia, and YbF_3, at a weight/volume ratio of 64.5/42.5 wt%/vol%.

Table 1. Components of resin systems for dental resin composites (DRCs).

DRC Experimental Groups	Components (wt%)					
	UDMA	Bis-EFMA	TEGDMA	CQ	DMAEMA	Fillers
UBT/Filler (30/70)	10.65	7.10	11.83	0.21	0.21	70
UBT/Filler (28/72)	9.94	6.62	11.04	0.20	0.20	72
UBT/Filler (26/74)	9.23	6.15	10.26	0.18	0.18	74
UBT/Filler (24/76)	8.52	5.68	9.46	0.17	0.17	76

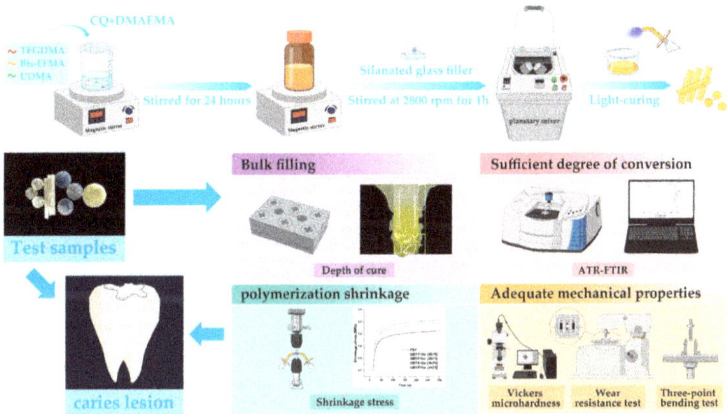

Figure 2. Schematic diagram of the preparation and testing of DRCs.

2.3. The Mixing Degree

After being subjected to light curing, the DRCs were deliberately fractured in liquid nitrogen to reveal their internal structure. Following the application of a gold coating, the extent of mixing between the resin matrix and inorganic fillers was meticulously examined on the newly exposed cross-section using a high-resolution scanning electron microscope (SEM; Merlin, Zeiss, Germany) operating at a voltage of 5 kV. This allowed for a detailed analysis of the composite's microstructure.

2.4. Double-Bond Conversion (DC)

Double-bond conversion of the BF-DRCs modified with different filler contents was evaluated by attenuated total reflection Fourier transform infrared spectroscopy (ATR-FTIR; Thermo Scientific Nicolet iS50, Thermo Fisher Scientific Inc., Waltham, MA, USA) using an attenuated total reflectance device with a diamond crystal. The uncured resin composite sample was filled into a cylindrical silicon mold with thicknesses of 2 mm, 3 mm, 4 mm, and 5 mm, and a diameter of 5 mm. Infrared light emitted from a source scanned the samples from the bottom to the top within a range of 4000 cm^{-1} to 400 cm^{-1}, with 4 scans measured per sample (resolution: 4 cm^{-1}). Based on the normalized peak area of the characteristic absorbance peaks associated with the polymerizable groups on the resin monomers, the DC of the ATR-FTIR spectra for samples with different thicknesses was evaluated using Equation (1):

$$\mathrm{DC}(\%) = \left[1 - \frac{(A_{C=C}/A_{C=O})_t}{(A_{C=C}/A_{C=O})_0}\right] \times 100 \quad (1)$$

In the absorption spectrum, $A_{C=C}$ at 1640 cm^{-1} and $A_{C=O}$ at 1720 cm^{-1} correspond to the peak areas of the characteristic and standard peaks (as shown in Figure 3). The subscripts t and 0 correspond to irradiation times of 40 s and 0 s (uncured state), respectively.

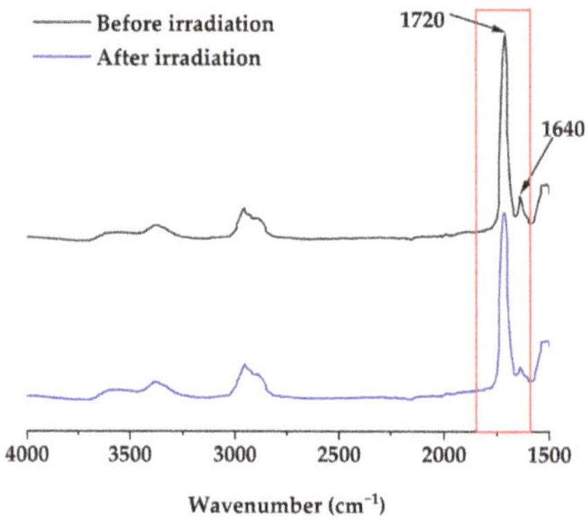

Figure 3. ATR-FTIR spectra of DRCs before and after irradiation at 1636 and 1720 cm^{-1}.

2.5. Depth of Cure (DOC)

DOC was measured following the method noted in ISO 4049:2019(E) [26]. The uncured samples were filled into a cylindrical stainless-steel mold, which had a diameter of 4 mm and a height of 15 mm. After 20 s and 40 s of light exposure, the samples were removed, and their uncured bottoms were scraped off with a plastic scraper. The height of the cured portion of the resin was measured using a spiral micrometer, and half of the measurement was taken as DOC.

2.6. Vickers Microhardness (VHN)

Cylindrical stainless-steel molds, with an inner diameter of 7 mm and heights ranging incrementally from 2 mm to 5 mm, were utilized to prepare the samples for VHN testing. All samples were irradiated from above for 40 s and subsequently stored in darkness at room temperature for 24 h before testing.

A Vickers microhardness tester (model HL-101, manufactured by Dongguan Magnanimity Instrument Equipment Co., Ltd. in Dongguan, China) was employed to measure the VHN of the DRC samples. To ensure accurate results, three samples from each group were tested, and for each sample, both the top and bottom surfaces were examined. Three random positions were selected and tested around the center of the cured sample at each surface level to account for potential variations in VHN and the crosslinking density across the specimen's surface. A load of 500 gf (with a dwell time of 5 s) was applied at each position, and the mean VHN value per surface level was determined from the three readings obtained. The ratio of the initial VHN values at the bottom and top surfaces was calculated to assess the depth-dependent effectiveness of the curing process [27].

2.7. Volumetric Shrinkage (VS)

Volumetric polymerization shrinkage was assessed by measuring density changes using Archimedes' principle. All the samples were weighed several times in two different environments of recognized density (conventional air and distilled water). Uncured samples were contained in 5 mL glass cups to facilitate density measurement. Equation (2) determined the density of the pre-photopolymerized sample (ρ_{ps}), the density of the empty cup (ρ_{ec}), and the overall density of the cup containing the uncured sample (ρ_{cc}):

$$\rho = \frac{m_a}{m_w - m_a}\rho_T \quad (2)$$

where ρ, m_w, m_a, and ρ_T are the density of the sample, weight of the sample in water, weight of the sample in air, and density of water at the measured temperature. The density of the uncured sample (ρ_{us}) was determined using Equation (3):

$$\rho_{\text{us}} = \frac{m_{\text{cca}} - m_{\text{eca}}}{\frac{m_{\text{cca}}}{\rho_{\text{cc}}} - \frac{m_{\text{eca}}}{\rho_{\text{ec}}}} \quad (3)$$

where ρ_{uc}, m_{cca}, m_{eca}, ρ_{cc}, and ρ_{ec} are the density of the uncured sample, the weight of the cup containing the uncured sample in air, the weight of the empty cup in air, the density of the cup containing the uncured sample, and the density of the empty cup.

Volume shrinkage (VS) can be calculated according to Equation (4), where ρ_{us} and ρ_{ps} are the sample density before and 40 s after photopolymerization:

$$\text{VS}(\%) = \left(1 - \frac{\rho_{\text{us}}}{\rho_{\text{ps}}}\right)100 \quad (4)$$

2.8. Shrinkage Stress (SS)

To measure the polymerization shrinkage stress (SS) of DRCs, two cylindrical glass fiber rods, each with a diameter of 6 mm and a length of 4 cm, were securely fastened in the universal testing machine (Z010, Zwick-Roell GmbH & Co. KG, Ulm, Germany) using a gripping device. Both ends of the rods were ensured to be uniformly flat and lightly coated with a layer of adhesive. The uncured resin composite was then carefully filled into the 1 mm gap between the rods, and any excess resin that squeezed out was scraped away. Two curing lamps, positioned 5 mm away from the resin composite on both sides, were used to irradiate the sample vertically for 20 s, simultaneously. At room temperature, the polymerization shrinkage force of the resin composite was measured and recorded for 300 s, generating a curve that depicted the variation in the force over time, along with the maximum polymerization shrinkage force value. The method for calculating the polymerization shrinkage stress is outlined in Equation (5):

$$\text{SS(MPa)} = \frac{4F_{\text{max}}}{\pi d^2} \quad (5)$$

where F_{max} (N) signifies the peak load encountered during the testing phase, whereas d (mm) indicates the diameter of the glass fiber rod. For each DRC, the above procedure was repeated five times.

2.9. Flexural Strength (FS) and Flexural Modulus (FM)

FS was assessed using the three-point bending test. Rectangular samples, measuring 2 mm × 2 mm × 25 mm, were utilized for this analysis, adhering to the ISO 4049:2019(E) [26] standard. Each group comprised twenty samples. Ten samples remained dry before testing, while the remaining samples were immersed in 35 mL of distilled water at 37 ± 1 °C until evaluation. A universal testing machine (AGS-10KN, Shimadzu Corporation, Kyoto, Japan) conducted the measurements at the speed of 1 mm/min. During the process, the FM of elasticity was also evaluated. According to ISO 4049 [26], DRCs were required to exhibit an FS of 80 MPa to comply with the criteria for restorative materials.

2.10. Water Sorption (WS) and Solubility (SL)

To evaluate WS and SL, the samples were prepared using silicone molds (15 mm diameter and 1 mm width). We applied tested materials in a single layer and irradiated them in nine non-overlapping zones, adhering to ISO 4049:2019(E) [26]. Eight samples were prepared for each DRC, stored in a desiccator to eliminate moisture, and their weight was recorded (FA1104J, Shunyuhengping Scientific Instrument Co., Ltd., Shanghai, China) at regular intervals until we achieved a constant mass (m_1). Dried samples were weighed (m_1) on a digital scale, which offered a minimum precision of 0.1 mg. After immersing them in 30 mL of distilled water at (37 ± 1) °C for 7 days, we weighed the samples' mass (m_2). Next, we dried the samples at 80 °C until their mass stabilized (m_3). WS and SL were calculated according to Equations (6) and (7):

$$\mathrm{WS}\left(\mu g/mm^3\right) = \frac{m_2 - m_1}{V} \tag{6}$$

$$\mathrm{SL}\left(\mu g/mm^3\right) = \frac{m_1 - m_3}{V} \tag{7}$$

where m_1 represents the initial mass of the sample, m_2 denotes the mass of the sample after water sorption, m_3 indicates the mass of the dried sample post-soaking, and V signifies the initial volume of the dried sample.

2.11. Wear Resistance

The MFT-4000 multifunctional material surface performance tester (MFT-4000, Lanzhou Huahui Instrument Technology Co., Lanzhou, China) facilitated reciprocating friction and wear assessments of DRC sample surfaces in ambient air conditions. The sample dimensions were 15 mm in width and 4 mm in height, polished on a water mill with 3000 grit silicon carbide sandpaper at a speed of 120 rpm for 30 min. This process ensured that both the top and bottom surfaces were parallel, smooth, and free of visible scratches. Subsequently, these samples were mounted on a high-speed reciprocating wear resistance testing machine, exposing the sample surface to reciprocating friction. ZrO_2 ceramic balls, with a 4 mm diameter and hardness akin to human teeth, were utilized as the friction pair. Modeling the normal chewing process in the oral cavity—with saliva serving as a lubricant—the chewing force was set between 3 and 36 N [28]. The load was established at 25 N, with a reciprocating speed of 200 mm/min and a length of 5 mm, all while maintaining ambient air conditions as the friction medium. Each sample underwent testing for 60 min. After the experiment, an optical profilometer (RTEC UP Dual Model, Rudolph Technologies, Inc., Wilmington, MA, USA) assessed the surface morphology, depth, and volume of grooves for each sample group under a 20× microscope.

2.12. Measurement of Cytotoxicity

We prepared the cell culture medium following ISO 10993-5 standards [29]. We incorporated 10% fetal bovine serum and 1% penicillin/streptomycin (100 units per milliliter) into the MEM basic medium (Gibco, Thermo Fisher Scientific, Waltham, MA, USA). Next, we fabricated cylindrical samples measuring 10 mm in diameter and 1 mm in height for each DRC. We then sterilized all samples by exposing them to UV light on each side for 1 h, then immersed them in the designated cell culture medium with a specific surface area to medium volume ratio of 1.25 cm^2/mL. Samples were stored in a 37 °C incubator for 24 h, filtered through a 0.22 μm sterile filter, and subsequently transferred to −4 °C for preservation. We cultivated L-929 mouse fibroblast cells (ICell-M026, Guangzhou Yanshi Technology Co., Ltd., Guangzhou, China) in a cell culture incubator at 37 °C under 5% CO_2 humidified air. A trypsin substitute (Tryp^{TM} Express, Thermo Fisher Scientific, USA) was used to dissociate the cells; then, we placed them on a 96-well plate at a density of 6000 cells per well, using a medium volume of 100 μL per well. After 24 h of incubation, the experimental group's medium was replaced with the sample extract, applying three concentration gradients of the extract: 100%, 50%, and 25% (diluted with cell culture medium), while the control group's medium was replaced with fresh cell culture medium as a negative control. This was followed by a 24 h incubation in the 37 °C cell culture incubator before evaluating cell viability using the Cell Counting Kit-8 (CCK-8, Dojindo Molecular Technology, Tokyo, Japan). After administering 10 μL of CCK-8 to each well, the samples were incubated for 2 h, then the absorbance was measured at 450 nm with a microplate reader (BioTek EPOCH$_2$, BioTek Instruments, Inc., Winooski, VT, USA). We calculated cell viability (CV) using Equation (8):

$$\mathrm{CV}(\%) = \frac{OD_e - OD_b}{OD_c - OD_b} \times 100 \tag{8}$$

where OD_e indicates the absorbance of the well containing treated cells exposed to the extract and CCK-8. OD_b represents the absorbance of the well containing only medium and CCK-8. Lastly, OD_c shows the absorbance of the well with untreated cells incubated in the medium with CCK-8.

2.13. Statistical Analysis

The statistical analysis of all data was conducted using SPSS 26.0 (IBM SPSS Statistics 26.0.0.0, Chicago, IL, USA). For inter-group data analysis, one-way analysis of variance (ANOVA) and Tukey's post hoc comparison test were employed to assess statistical differences between groups, with $p < 0.05$ indicating significant differences. When the number of samples between groups was less than three, an independent samples T-test was utilized, and after verifying homogeneity of variance, $p < 0.05$ also indicated significant differences.

3. Results

This electron microscope analysis revealed that all inorganic filler particles and resin matrix added to the BF-DRCs were successfully combined in different DRCs, as shown in Figure 4.

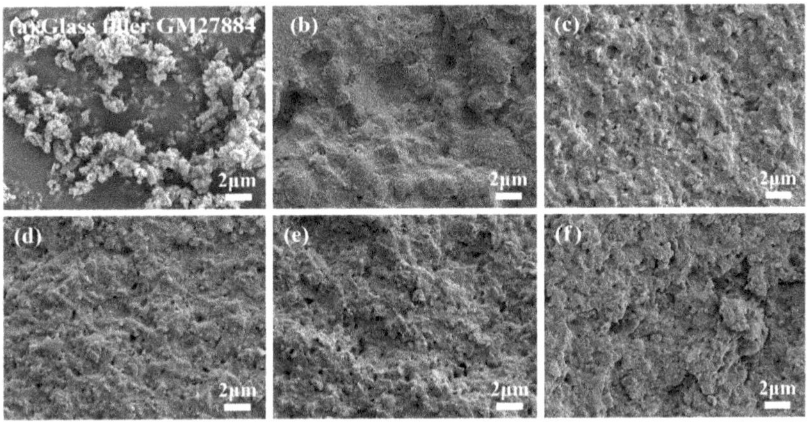

Figure 4. SEM images depict the micro-filler particles utilized as additional fillers for BF-DRCs: (**a**) SCHOTT® UltraFine silanated inorganic glass fillers, and the section morphology of DRCs: (**b**) DRCs of FBF, (**c**) DRCs of UBT/Filler (30/70), (**d**) DRCs of UBT/Filler (28/72), (**e**) DRCs of UBT/Filler (26/74), and (**f**) DRCs of UBT/Filler (24/76).

The results for DOC, WS, and SL are shown in Table 2. We can notice how UBT/Filler (30/70) and UBT/Filler (24/76) presented a deeper depth of cure (40 s) compared to FBF, with an average DOC of 5.589 mm in a range between 5.389 and 5.789 mm for UBT/Filler (30/70) and a mean value of 5.660 mm in a range between 5.460 and 5.860 mm for UBT/Filler (24/76). There was no significant change in the DOC of the experimental groups with increasing filler content when the curing time was extended from 20 s to 40 s ($p > 0.05$). The WS of the experimental groups presented a significant decrease ($p < 0.05$) with increasing filler content, and there was no significant difference in SL ($p > 0.05$). The commercial control FBF had no significant difference in DOC (20 s) over the experimental group ($p > 0.05$), while the FBF had higher WS and SL ($p < 0.05$).

Mean values and standard deviations of VHN registered with the samples (thicknesses of 2, 3, 4, and 5 mm) for the top and bottom surfaces are listed in Table 3. We considered the five bulk-fill dental resin composites (FBF, UBT/Filler (30/70), UBT/Filler (28/72), UBT/Filler (26/74), and UBT/Filler (24/76)) and compared their hardness ratios, in accordance with the external (top) versus the internal side (bottom) of the samples, as shown in Table 3. Despite decreased values observed between the top and bottom surfaces with increased sample thicknesses, the hardness ratio exceeded 0.80 across all groups. Statistical analysis of variance (ANOVA) showed that all experimental groups had a significant VHN increase ($p < 0.05$) with the increasing filler content, under the same thickness of sample conditions. With the proportion of 24/76 (UBT/Filler), it showed much higher ($p < 0.05$) VHN than FBF regardless of thicknesses.

Table 2. Depth of cure (DOC) of DRCs (curing time = 20 s and 40 s), as well as water sorption (WS) and solubility (SL) of DRCs (curing time = 40 s).

DRCs	DOC (mm) $n = 6$		WS and SL (μg/mm^3) $n = 6$	
	DOC_{20s} (mm) ($p = 0.451$)	DOC_{40s} (mm) ($p = 0.011$)	WS (μg/mm^3) ($p = 0.000$)	SL (μg/mm^3) ($p = 0.000$)
FBF	4.197 ± 0.1^{a}	5.018 ± 0.2^{b}	33.27 ± 1.8^{a}	13.65 ± 1.9^{a}
UBT/Filler (30/70)	4.289 ± 0.1^{a}	5.589 ± 0.2^{a}	24.27 ± 1.3^{b}	6.53 ± 0.7^{b}
UBT/Filler (28/72)	4.290 ± 0.3^{a}	$5.427 \pm 0.3^{a,b}$	25.74 ± 2.2^{b}	6.81 ± 1.1^{b}
UBT/Filler (26/74)	4.194 ± 0.2^{a}	$5.398 \pm 0.3^{a,b}$	21.53 ± 0.2^{c}	5.79 ± 1.1^{b}
UBT/Filler (24/76)	4.415 ± 0.2^{a}	5.660 ± 0.2^{a}	21.66 ± 1.3^{c}	5.76 ± 1.1^{b}

[a,b,c] Different lowercase superscript letters indicate differences within the same column ($p < 0.05$).

Table 3. Vickers microhardness (VHN) of DRCs (curing time = 40 s).

Height, mm	DRCs	VHN $n = 9$				
		Top ($HV_{0.5}$)	p-Value	Bottom ($HV_{0.5}$)	p-Value	Bottom/Top (%)
2	FBF	61.4 ± 0.2^{a}	$p = 0.000$	58.4 ± 1.2^{b}	$p = 0.000$	95.2
	UBT/Filler (30/70)	51.3 ± 1.3^{c}		50.3 ± 0.7^{d}		98.0
	UBT/Filler (28/72)	52.4 ± 0.5^{c}		51.3 ± 0.9^{d}		97.9
	UBT/Filler (26/74)	55.6 ± 1.2^{b}		55.6 ± 1.2^{c}		100.0
	UBT/Filler (24/76)	62.6 ± 1.4^{a}		62.1 ± 1.7^{a}		99.2
3	FBF	60.0 ± 1.2^{b}	$p = 0.000$	58.9 ± 1.2^{b}	$p = 0.000$	98.1
	UBT/Filler (30/70)	49.6 ± 0.3^{e}		50.2 ± 1.3^{c}		101.2
	UBT/Filler (28/72)	53.4 ± 2.0^{d}		52.1 ± 1.5^{c}		97.5
	UBT/Filler (26/74)	57.1 ± 0.5^{c}		58.6 ± 1.5^{b}		102.6
	UBT/Filler (24/76)	63.2 ± 1.6^{a}		63.6 ± 0.1^{a}		100.7
4	FBF	60.0 ± 1.2^{b}	$p = 0.000$	55.7 ± 0.7^{b}	$p = 0.000$	92.9
	UBT/Filler (30/70)	49.6 ± 0.6^{e}		49.3 ± 0.9^{d}		99.2
	UBT/Filler (28/72)	54.2 ± 1.1^{d}		52.0 ± 1.5^{c}		95.9
	UBT/Filler (26/74)	57.8 ± 1.6^{c}		56.7 ± 0.6^{b}		98.1
	UBT/Filler (24/76)	63.6 ± 0.1^{a}		63.4 ± 0.8^{a}		99.7
5	FBF	60.9 ± 1.7^{b}	$p = 0.000$	51.0 ± 2.8^{c}	$p = 0.000$	83.8
	UBT/Filler (30/70)	49.5 ± 0.7^{d}		46.9 ± 0.9^{b}		94.9
	UBT/Filler (28/72)	52.4 ± 0.7^{c}		50.7 ± 0.7^{c}		96.7
	UBT/Filler (26/74)	58.7 ± 2.8^{b}		56.7 ± 0.5^{b}		96.6
	UBT/Filler (24/76)	63.9 ± 1.0^{a}		63.9 ± 1.0^{a}		100.0

[a–e] Different lowercase superscript letters indicate differences within the same column of the same thicknesses ($p < 0.05$).

Mean values and standard deviations of DC results of the samples at different thicknesses (thicknesses of 2, 3, 4, and 5 mm) are listed in Table 4. The DC of DRCs in the experimental groups with different filler content was not significantly different at each sample thickness ($p > 0.05$). When the thickness of all DRC samples was increased to 5 mm, the DC decreased significantly, except for UBT/Filler (30/70; $p < 0.05$).

Table 4. Double-bond conversion (DC) of DRCs (curing time = 40 s).

DRCs	DC (%)				
	2 mm (p = 0.000)	3 mm (p = 0.007)	4 mm (p = 0.000)	5 mm (p = 0.000)	p-Value
FBF	48.7 ± 1.7 ^{b,A}	46.7 ± 1.9 ^{b,A}	32.6 ± 7.7 ^{b,A}	32.8 ± 2.1 ^{b,A}	p = 0.092
UBT/Filler (30/70)	53.4 ± 1.9 ^{a,A}	53.5 ± 3.0 ^{a,A}	52.3 ± 4.4 ^{a,A}	51.3 ± 2.5 ^{a,A}	p = 0.743
UBT/Filler (28/72)	56.1 ± 1.0 ^{a,A}	52.9 ± 2.6 ^{a,A,B}	53.5 ± 3.5 ^{a,A,B}	50.1 ± 3.5 ^{a,B}	p = 0.042
UBT/Filler (26/74)	55.2 ± 1.5 ^{a,A}	55.9 ± 2.6 ^{a,A}	53.0 ± 3.0 ^{a,A,B}	50.1 ± 2.4 ^{a,B}	p = 0.013
UBT/Filler (24/76)	55.3 ± 1.0 ^{a,A}	52.8 ± 2.7 ^{a,A,B}	49.6 ± 2.3 ^{a,B}	48.5 ± 4.0 ^{a,B}	p = 0.005

^{a,b} Different lowercase superscript letters indicate differences within the same column of the same thicknesses ($p < 0.05$). ^{A,B} Different capitalized superscript letters indicate differences between thicknesses of the same sample ($p < 0.05$).

The tested materials' mean SS (±SD), expressed in MPa, as well as mean VS (±SD) are shown in Table 5. Representative SS versus time curves are shown in Figure 5. The statistical analysis of variance for SS evaluation showed that FBF presented significantly lower stress during irradiation than the other tested materials ($p < 0.05$). For the experimental groups, no significant difference in the SS values of the DRCs was observed with the increasing filler content ($p > 0.05$). The VS of all experimental groups decreased with the increase in filler in the resin system ($p < 0.05$). UBT/Filler (26/74) and UBT/Filler (24/76) showed much lower ($p < 0.05$) VS than FBF. Figure 5 illustrates that the SS of all DRCs initially increased rapidly and then gradually leveled off. However, during the first 20 s, as the inorganic filler content in the system increased, the initial increase rate of DRC curing accelerated significantly, and except for UBT/Filler (30/70), the final SS showed a notable upward trend.

Table 5. Shrinkage stress (SS) and volumetric shrinkage (VS) of DRCs.

DRCs	SS (MPa) (p = 0.002)	VS (%) (p = 0.009)
FBF	1.60 ± 0.1 ^{b}	4.91 ± 0.3 ^{a,b}
UBT/Filler (30/70)	2.05 ± 0.2 ^{a}	5.08 ± 0.6 ^{a}
UBT/Filler (28/72)	1.93 ± 0.2 ^{a}	4.86 ± 0.5 ^{a,b}
UBT/Filler (26/74)	2.05 ± 0.2 ^{a}	4.80 ± 0.8 ^{b}
UBT/Filler (24/76)	2.16 ± 0.3 ^{a}	4.65 ± 0.6 ^{b}

^{a,b} Different lowercase superscript letters indicate differences within the same column ($p < 0.05$).

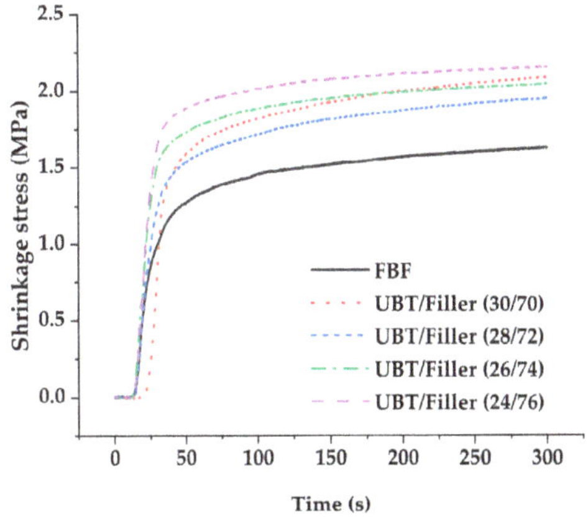

Figure 5. Shrinkage stress versus time curves of DRCs.

The mean and standard deviation results for FS and FM of each DRC following different storage conditions are shown in Figure 6. Following each storage condition, the FBF appeared to be significantly stronger since it showed the greatest FS values in contrast to all BF-DRCs ($p < 0.05$). In addition, the FM of the FBF was considerably higher than all BF-DRCs following each storage condition ($p < 0.05$). For the experimental groups, the FS in each group did not change significantly with the increase in the filler content ($p > 0.05$). The FM increased with the increasing filler content ($p < 0.05$), and the FM of the UBT/Filler (30/70) and UBT/Filler (26/74) had no significant difference before and after water immersion ($p > 0.05$). All tested DRCs met the performance requirements of achieving 80 MPa FS, as stipulated by ISO 4049 [26].

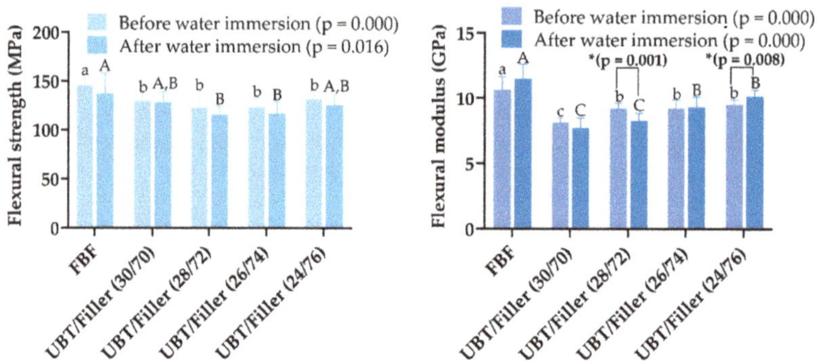

Figure 6. Flexural strength and modulus before and after water immersion of DRCs. [a,b,c] Different lowercase superscript letters indicate differences in FS or FM before water immersion with the same composition and proportion ($p < 0.05$). [A,B,C] Different capital superscript letters indicate differences in FS or FM after water immersion with the same composition and proportion ($p < 0.05$). * Asterisk indicates a significant difference between before and after water immersion ($p < 0.05$). Bar graphs were created using GraphPad Prism 9.5.

The volume wear results for the five resin materials are illustrated in Figure 7a. FBF demonstrated significantly higher volume wear ($p < 0.05$), whereas the other groups showed no significant difference ($p > 0.05$). The depth and morphology of all DRCs, examined through optical profilometry following the wear resistance test, are displayed in Figure 7b–f. Under the same friction load and cycles, FBF exhibited deeper and wider indentations. In contrast, the experimental groups showed shallower and lighter indentations. Increasing the filler content from UBT/Filler (30/70) to UBT/Filler (24/76) resulted in a slight rise in volumetric abrasion, yet this change lacked statistical significance ($p > 0.05$).

Figure 8 shows the results of the CCK-8 assay. The cell viability of all DRCs was greater than 70% at 100%, 50%, and 25% extract concentrations.

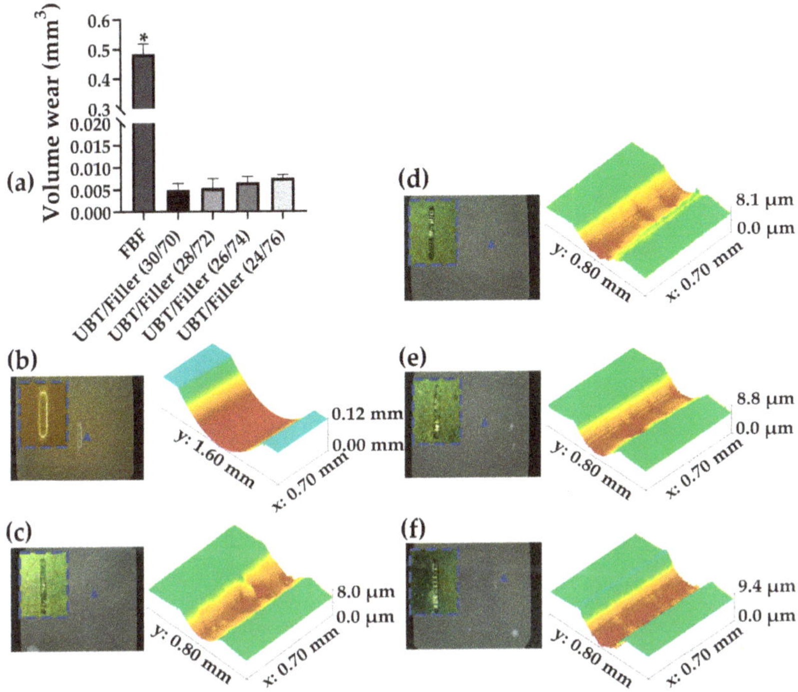

Figure 7. (**a**) Volume wear of dental resin composites ($p = 0.000$). (**b**–**f**) Surface morphology (triangle annotation) and 3D profile scanning images (20×) of samples after wear testing. The image within the dashed box shows an enlarged view of the wear marks at the triangular identifier. (**b**) DRCs of FBF, (**c**) DRCs of UBT/Filler (30/70), (**d**) DRCs of UBT/Filler (28/72), (**e**) DRCs of UBT/Filler (26/74), and (**f**) DRCs of UBT/Filler (24/76). * Asterisk indicates a significant difference between different groups ($p < 0.05$). Bar graphs were created using GraphPad Prism 9.5.

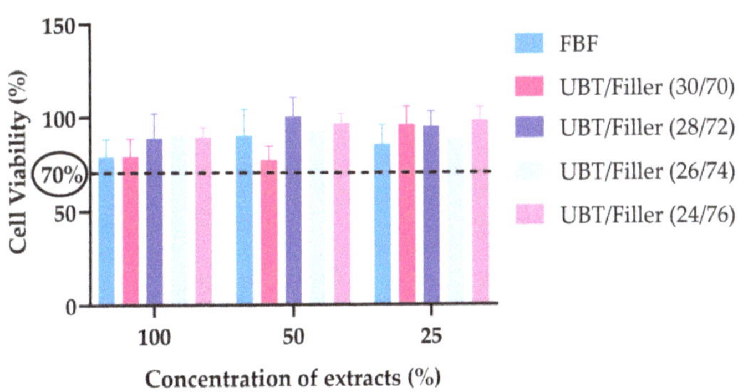

Figure 8. Cell viability of DRCs (100%, 50%, and 25% extract). The dashed line indicates that cell activity has reached 70%. Bar graphs were created using GraphPad Prism 9.5.

4. Discussion

DOC is a key parameter of DRCs, directly impacting their curing effectiveness. A notable feature of BF-DRC is its ability to deliver incremental fillings of 4 mm to 5 mm in a single treatment session, thereby reducing the clinical operation time [30]. Insufficient curing depth can cause more material to leach from poorly cured resin at the base of the filling, potentially irritating soft tissues and dental pulp, promoting bacterial growth, and triggering allergic reactions [31]. Enhancing the translucency of BF-DRCs is a crucial strategy for optimizing the curing process. The translucency of DRCs is influenced by the amount of filler and the refractive index variation between the filler particles and the resin matrix [32]. This disparity determines the extent of light penetration within the DRC. When the particle size of the filler is uniform, increasing the filler content generally leads to reduced translucency, a finding supported by most literature in this area [19,33]. Studies indicate that BF-DRCs with a lower filler content display significantly higher DOC than conventional DRCs, likely due to the minimal filler quantity aiding in polymerization and light transmission, thereby improving curing at greater depths [20]. In this study, the DOC of different materials was assessed using the scraping method described in ISO 4049. Under irradiation with a 550 mW/cm^2 LED unit for 20 or 40 s, the tested DRCs met the standards for DOC in bulk-filled dental resin composites, all exceeding 4 mm. Additionally, the increased filler content did not significantly affect the DOC in the experimental group, leading to the rejection of the first null hypothesis.

Various alternative techniques, such as Vickers microhardness testing and infrared spectroscopy, can assess the DOC. Furthermore, it has been suggested that the ISO 4049 [26] scratch method may overstate the DOC [34]. Numerous studies have shown that the light transmittance of DRC shows a positive correlation with the VHN ratio of the bottom-to-top layers, suggesting a significant relationship between VHN and DOC [35,36]. In this study, the VHN bottom/top ratio of the 4 mm-thick DRC sample exceeded 80%, indicating that the tested sample meets the curing depth requirements for BF-DRCs [37]. Some DRCs exhibited bottom/top values greater than 100% at smaller thicknesses. This phenomenon may be attributed to the presence of an oxygen inhibition layer on the surface of the DRCs. Although a polyester film was employed during sample preparation to minimize atmospheric oxygen exposure, some oxygen may still affect the surface layer by generating radicals that can bond with resin monomers. These oxygen radicals can create stable peroxide radicals and are non-reactive, leading to incomplete polymerization of monomers on the resin surface, thus forming an oxygen-inhibition layer [38]. These factors subsequently impact the VHN at the surface of the DRCs. Moreover, this may relate to the post-curing of the samples, as flexible chains in the resin system can continue to polymerize at a certain rate for a short period after stopping the light exposure. The number of free radicals participating in post-curing at the sample bottom is significantly higher than at the top, making it difficult for the hardness ratio between the bottom and top to reflect the true curing effect. Reports indicate that the hardness of DRCs shows a significant improvement after 24 h of curing compared to 15 min, aligning with theoretical predictions of polymerization following irradiation within the resin [39].

VHN characterizes the resistance of DRCs to plastic deformation and wear. Research shows that the VHN of DRCs is influenced by the type, morphology, size, and content of filler particles. Increasing the filler content results in a higher VHN [40]. El-Safty et al. [41] investigated the nano-hardness of ten types of DRCs using nano-indentation, discovering a positive correlation between the nano-hardness of this series of resin composites and the filler loading. Jun et al. [42] studied 18 different DRCs to explore the relationship between the mechanical properties of various resin composite and filler fractions. They found that the surface hardness increased with the filler content, particularly when the filler particles were silanized, resulting in a significant increase in the hardness values of the DRCs with rising filler fractions. In this study, the increase in the content of inorganic fillers increased the VHN of the DRC, which further confirmed this view.

The polymerization process is intrinsically linked to the monomer chemistry, filler characteristics, photo-initiator concentration, and polymerization conditions [43]. Since the polymerization conditions, layer thickness, curing unit strength, and exposure time were standardized in this study, differences in the DC value of DRCs can be attributed to the different compositions of the materials, mostly to variations in the chemistry of their resin matrix and the filler loading. Research indicates that the DC decreased with an increase in the content of opaque fillers [44]. Higher DC values for DRC indicated lower levels of unreacted monomers within the resin composite and less cytotoxicity to the repair produced, with current resin composites having a final DC in the range of 50% to 80% [45]. The experiment revealed that the commercial control dental resin composite FBF possessed the lowest DC value. In contrast, the experimental groups (UBT/Filler system) demonstrated a higher DC, while no direct correlation was found between DC and filler content within the experimental groups. The variation in DC values might be more closely related to the chemical composition of the resin matrix, initial viscosity, and the flexibility of the monomer's crystalline structure [46]. As the thickness of all DRC samples increased, a significant decline in DC was observed. This decrease occurred because the resin composite's polymerization process was initiated by visible light, and the scattering of light by filler particles influenced the depth of light penetration. When thickness increments of 4–5 mm were applied, the effectiveness of the photo-initiator decreased in deeper regions due to light intensity attenuation, subsequently affecting the system's polymerization and DC value. With an increase in inorganic filler content, the viscosity of the system rose, limiting the activity of high-molecular-weight free radicals, thereby restricting the chain growth step and leading to a decrease in DC value [47]. DC significantly impacts the mechanical properties and biocompatibility of DRCs. A high DC correlates with high polymerization shrinkage, while a low conversion rate relates to low mechanical performance, poor color stability, and reduced biocompatibility [45,48]. The testing of DC also provides data support for subsequent performance analysis.

Ideally, DRCs should exhibit high stability and waterproof characteristics. Water absorption emerges as a critical property influencing the clinical success of resin composite. It negatively impacts the hydrolytic stability of these materials, leading to discoloration [48], degradation of mechanical properties, reduced wear resistance, and hydrolytic degradation at the resin–filler interface [49]. WS and SL occur primarily when resin composites are exposed to aqueous environments, such as the oral cavity, allowing them to absorb water and release unreacted monomers. They are, therefore, related to the DC of the DRC; the higher the DC, the lower the number of unreacted monomers, leading to lower WS and SL values, while factors such as the type of monomer, filler content, and type also affect them [50]. The experimental data indicated that an increase in filler content contributed to a reduction in the water sorption (WS) of DRCs in the UBT/Filler system. Excluding the effects of DC, this reduction may relate to the water absorption capacity associated with the available equilibrium pore volume and the hydrophilicity of the resin monomers. As the inorganic filler content in resin composites increased, the concentration of hydrophilic resin monomers in the corresponding materials decreased, leading to an overall decline in WS. FBF exhibited higher WS and SL, likely due to its lower monomer conversion rate and the presence of smaller nanoparticle fillers, possessed a larger surface area, and could absorb more water. Likewise, smaller filler particles enhanced the filler/matrix interface area, increasing the resin composite's susceptibility to water penetration and degradation [51].

VS during polymerization and the formation of interfacial gaps remain issues affecting the longevity of resin composite restorations. It is an unavoidable property of the polymerization process due to the short covalent bonds that result in a decrease in the distance between the monomer molecules, which reduces the total free volume within the monomer structure and produces a dense buildup of polymer molecules [52]. The size of the VS generates shrinkage stress, which affects the bonding interface between the tooth and the restoration. When the induced stress exceeds the adhesive strength between the bonding agent and the tooth, interfacial gaps will form [53]. Bis-EFMA-based BF-DRC achieves the purpose of reducing polymerization shrinkage by reducing the percentage of short double bonds through higher molecular weight. Experimental data indicated that the VS of DRCs in the UBT/Filler system decreased as the content of inorganic fillers increased. This trend may arise because the inorganic fillers maintain a constant volume before and after polymerization. Consequently, DRCs with a higher content of inorganic fillers exhibited lower VS under a given volume. SS arises from the shrinkage of DRCs under constrained conditions. This stress can lead to micro-gaps forming, resulting in micro-leakage of saliva and bacteria, degradation of the adhesive interface, secondary caries, pulpal changes, and ultimately clinical failure of restorations [54,55]. However, SS is not only related to the VS and DC of the DRCs but is also significantly associated with the elastic modulus during the formation of the polymer network [56,57]. Studies have evaluated the SS and elastic modulus of different BF-DRCs. They found that the SS of DRCs correlates with the composition of monomers and filler content. In addition, there is a notable correlation between SS and elastic modulus: a lower elastic modulus can facilitate stress dissipation during polymerization, while a higher elastic modulus can lead to higher shrinkage stress, even in low-shrinkage composites [58]. Figure 5 shows that the SS of UBT/Filler (24/76) and UBT/Filler (30/70) was high, likely linked to the system's VS and FM. The high FM of UBT/Filler (24/76) hindered the dissipation of stress generated during polymerization [59], while the greater SS of UBT/Filler (30/70) was attributed to its higher VS. Reports indicate that SS positively correlates with the VS [60]. The differences between FBF and UBT/Filler systems stem from the distinct resin matrices and fillers used, which will not be discussed further in this paper. In conclusion, the increase in the inorganic powder filler content can significantly reduce the polymerization volume shrinkage of the system, so the third null hypothesis was rejected.

Extensive research has been conducted on FS and FM of DRCs to predict their performance in real clinical environments. Mechanical properties depend on factors such as the composition of the resin matrix, viscosity, and the type and content of fillers [61]. Studies indicate a correlation between the mechanical performance of DRCs and filler content [62,63]. Reports have assessed Bis-GMA/TEGDMA-based DRCs with filler loading levels ranging from 0 to 70 wt%. Research shows that the FM of DRCs increases exponentially with the rise in filler content. However, only minor differences in modulus were observed among DRCs containing 0–60 wt% fillers. In contrast, resins with 70 wt% fillers demonstrated significantly higher FM across all conversion levels [64]. It has also been reported that higher filler content does not always result in superior mechanical performance [65,66]. Fronza et al. characterized the effect of inorganic filler content in conventional DRCs (Herculite Classic, HER, 50 vol% filler content) and four types of BF-DRCs (Tetric EvoCeram Bulk Fill, TEC, 60 vol% filler content; Filtek Bulk Fill, FBF, 42.5 vol% filler content; EverX Posterior, EXP, 57 vol% filler content; Surefil SDR flow, SDR, 44 vol% filler content) on the biaxial flexural strength (FS) and flexural modulus (FM). The research found that although the FM of DRCs was influenced by filler mass fraction, the FS of EXP and TEC was lower than that of the lower-filler-loaded FBF and SDR [67]. The increase in polymer network density, stress transfer between filler particles and the resin matrix, and the adhesion between components also affected the degree of polymerization and the final performance of DRCs [68]. The experimental test results indicated that increasing the filler content did not have a significant impact on the FS of the UBT/Filler system. This was primarily because FS depends on the DC of DRCs rather than on the filler content or adequate silanization [69]. After immersion, the FS decreased slightly, but this difference was not statistically significant. Theoretically, prolonged soaking can impair the mechanical properties of the DRC. This deterioration occurs due to the degradation of the resin matrix, filler particles, or the silane layer at the interfaces. Water intrusion into the DRC may cause the hydrolytic breakdown of the silane layer, leading to debonding of filler particles and potentially their hydrolysis. The resin matrix swells and becomes plasticized upon water exposure. Thus, the flexural strength of the DRC will likely decline after soaking [50]. In this experiment, although the FS of the BF-DRCs decreased in numerical value after immersion, there was no statistically significant difference in FS before and after immersion. The increase in inorganic filler content significantly improved the FM of the DRC in the UBT/Filler system, a phenomenon supported by the theoretical analysis mentioned earlier [64]. The FM of UBT/Filler (28/72) significantly decreased before and after water immersion, possibly due to water molecules diffusing into the polymer network, functioning as a plasticizer, resulting in a decreased FM of DRCs. In contrast, the FM of UBT/Filler (24/76) increased significantly, while the higher filler contents in UBT/Filler (26/74) and FBF also showed an increasing trend in FM after immersion. This phenomenon may arise because the greater filler ratios in high- and medium-viscosity DRCs decrease the amount of resin vulnerable to water aging. Combined with the above, increasing the filler content could significantly improve the VHN and FM of Bis-EFMA-based BF-DRCs, so null hypothesis 2 was rejected.

Insufficient wear resistance of DRCs under chewing loads is a common reason for the premature failure of restorations. Generally, the variations in wear among the resin composite relate primarily to the volume and distribution of filler particles, the properties of the resin matrix, the degree of conversion, and the bonding between the resin matrix and filler [70]. It is theorized that DRCs with lower filler contents may exhibit higher wear values, as DRCs with higher filler contents have a greater surface Vickers hardness, which provides more protection to the resin matrix from filler abrasion, making the surface less susceptible to wear. However, Shimokawa et al. [71] revealed that DRCs with a high filler volume fraction showed more wear, while those with lower filler loadings experienced less. Hu et al. [72] investigated the fundamental wear behavior of resin composite with various filler contents under two-body wear conditions. Their study found that DRCs with a filler volume percentage below 60% had a lower two-body wear rate, while DRCs with a filler volume content of 80–87.5% exhibited higher wear rates. Under two-body wear conditions, incorporating highly loaded filler particles into the resin matrix decreased the wear resistance of DRCs. In this experiment, under the larger friction wear load of 25 N, the resin layer on the DRC surface, which is prone to damage, was rapidly worn away. This can lead to abrasion between the resin matrix and the exposed filler, with UBT/Filler (24/76), which has a higher filler content, experiencing more abrasion. In the current study, no significant relationship was found between filler content and wear amounts of DRCs, although the wear amounts across all experimental groups were notably lower than that of the commercial control FBF.

BF-DRCs are often employed for filling restorations in deeper cavities of posterior teeth due to their higher curing depth and other characteristics. Considering the unique features of the pulp–dentin complex, the filling materials must exhibit low cytotoxicity [73]. Ideally, DRCs should be non-toxic to both oral hard and soft tissues. However, numerous in vitro studies have indicated that the polymerization reaction of crosslinked polymer matrices generated by dimethacrylate resin monomers never completes 100%. The release of unpolymerized monomers can trigger cytotoxic reactions. In addition to the leaching of unreacted monomers, cytotoxicity may also stem from the release of initiators from the resin matrix or metal ions from inorganic fillers. This type of cytotoxic restorative material can elicit both short-term and long-term adverse tissue responses, ranging from postoperative sensitivity to irreversible pulp damage [73–75]. A study evaluated the cytotoxicity of flowable and paste-like BF-DRCs using real-time cell analysis, with conventional DRCs as a reference. The findings indicated that flowable and paste-like DRCs of the same brand exhibited similar cytotoxicity. Throughout the experiment, a significant reduction in cell viability was observed for BBF (Beautifil-Bulk Flowable) and BBR (Beautifil-Bulk Restorative). Considering that both DRCs contain pre-reacted glass-ionomer (PRG) fillers in their resin matrix, the higher fluoride release from PRG-filled DRCs compared to others suggests that the cytotoxicity of BBR and BBF may be linked to the fluoride and other metal ions released, such as aluminum, boron, sodium, silicon, strontium, and zinc, from the PRG fillers. This indicates that metal ions released from inorganic fillers in DRCs also significantly impact cytotoxicity [76]. Additionally, research has explored the correlation between filler content and the cytotoxicity of DRCs. Shajii et al. investigated the impact of inorganic filler content on the biodegradation of the Bis-GMA/TEGDMA resin system using cholesterol esterase. They found that the cumulative release of biodegradation products from DRC with 20 wt% filler was significantly higher than that from DRC with 40 wt% filler, indicating that the release of biodegradation products is related to the "filler/resin" ratio [77]. All the BF-DRCs involved in this study exhibited low cytotoxicity (with cell viability at 70% or higher), and no significant differences in cell viability were observed among the DRCs. Experimental data also indicated that the cell viability of FBF extracts was slightly lower than that of the UBT/Filler system. This difference may be attributed to the low solubility and high monomer conversion rate of the UBT/Filler system, resulting in a reduced release of unreacted monomers. The research demonstrated that an increase in inorganic filler content did not notably impact the cytotoxicity of BF-DRCs; however, considering that the variation in filler content within the system was minimal, the discussion on the effect of filler content on cytotoxicity remains limited. Overall, the UBT/Filler system exhibited lower cytotoxicity, indicating potential for clinical application as an oral restorative material.

5. Conclusions

Based on the results obtained in this study, the following conclusions were drawn:

1. The increase in inorganic filler content did not significantly affect the DOC, DC, SL, and cytotoxicity, and it could notably reduce the WS of the system of Bis-EFMA-based BF-DRCs.
2. The increase in inorganic filler content could significantly enhance the VHN and FM of Bis-EFMA-based BF-DRCs, aiding in the improvement of the mechanical properties of the system.
3. The increase in inorganic filler content could significantly reduce the VS of Bis-EFMA-based BF-DRC, to a certain extent, which could help improve the polymeric shrinkage of the system.
4. The UBT/Filler system with UBT/Filler (24/76) exhibited superior performance compared to commercial bulk-fill resin composite FBF in all aspects, except for flexural strength, flexural modulus, and polymerization shrinkage stress. While the flexural strength of UBT/Filler (24/76) was significantly lower than that of FBF, it still exceeded the minimum flexural strength requirement of 80 MPa, as stipulated by ISO 4049:2019(E), thereby meeting the mechanical performance criteria for posterior dental restorative materials.
5. Bis-EFMA-based BF-DRCs can achieve good operability, exceptional mechanical strength, and reduced polymerization shrinkage through an increase in filler content within a certain range. However, considering the prospects for clinical application, their biocompatibility requires further experimental discussion. Additionally, this study has limitations, such as testing the in vitro properties, which may not fully replicate the complexities of the oral environment. Moreover, the introduction of a single filler system cannot adequately balance the modulus of the system and polymerization shrinkage stress.

Author Contributions: H.D., writing—original draft, investigation, methodology, and formal analysis; F.L., writing—review and editing and supervision; J.H., writing—review and editing, conceptualization, methodology, and supervision. All authors have read and agreed to the published version of the manuscript.

Funding: This research received no external funding.

Institutional Review Board Statement: Not applicable.

Informed Consent Statement: Not applicable.

Data Availability Statement: The original contributions presented in the study are included in the article, further inquiries can be directed to the corresponding author/s.

Conflicts of Interest: The authors declare that they have no known competing financial interests or personal relationships that could have appeared to influence the work reported in this paper.

References

1. Miletic, V. *Dental Composite Materials for Direct Restorations*; Springer International Publishing: Cham, Switzerland, 2018.
2. Cho, K.; Rajan, G.; Farrar, P.; Prentice, L.; Prusty, B.G. Dental resin composites: A review on materials to product realizations. *Compos. Part B Eng.* **2022**, *230*, 109495. [CrossRef]

3. Van Landuyt, K.L.; Nawrot, T.; Geebelen, B.; De Munck, J.; Snauwaert, J.; Yoshihara, K.; Scheers, H.; Godderis, L.; Hoet, P.; Van Meerbeek, B.; et al. How much do resin-based dental materials release? A meta-analytical approach. *Dent. Mater.* **2011**, *27*, 723–747. [CrossRef]
4. De Nys, S.; Turkalj, M.; Duca, R.C.; Covaci, A.; Elskens, M.; Godderis, L.; Vanoirbeek, J.; Van Meerbeek, B.; Van Landuyt, K.L. Level of BPA contamination in resin composites determines BPA release. *Dent. Mater.* **2024**, *40*, 1025–1030. [CrossRef] [PubMed]
5. De Angelis, F.; Sarteur, N.; Buonvivere, M.; Vadini, M.; Šteffl, M.; D'Arcangelo, C. Meta-analytical analysis on components released from resin-based dental materials. *Clin. Oral Investig.* **2022**, *26*, 6015–6041. [CrossRef] [PubMed]
6. Roussou, K.; Nikolaidis, A.K.; Ziouti, F.; Arhakis, A.; Arapostathis, K.; Koulaouzidou, E.A. Cytotoxic Evaluation and Determination of Organic and Inorganic Eluates from Restorative Materials. *Molecules* **2021**, *26*, 4912. [CrossRef] [PubMed]
7. Snijder, C.A.; Heederik, D.; Pierik, F.H.; Hofman, A.; Jaddoe, V.W.; Koch, H.M.; Longnecker, M.P.; Burdorf, A. Fetal Growth and Prenatal Exposure to Bisphenol A: The Generation R Study. *Environ. Health Perspect.* **2013**, *121*, 393–398. [CrossRef] [PubMed]
8. Ejaredar, M.; Lee, Y.; Roberts, D.J.; Sauve, R.; Dewey, D. Bisphenol A exposure and children's behavior: A systematic review. *J. Expo. Sci. Environ. Epidemiol.* **2017**, *27*, 175–183. [CrossRef]
9. González-Casanova, J.E.; Bermúdez, V.; Fuentes, N.J.C.; Angarita, L.C.; Caicedo, N.H.; Muñoz, J.R.; Rojas-Gómez, D.M. New Evidence on BPA's Role in Adipose Tissue Development of Proinflammatory Processes and Its Relationship with Obesity. *Int. J. Mol. Sci.* **2023**, *24*, 8231. [CrossRef] [PubMed]
10. Hessel, E.V.; Ezendam, J.; van Broekhuizen, F.A.; Hakkert, B.; DeWitt, J.; Granum, B.; Guzylack, L.; Lawrence, B.P.; Penninks, A.; Rooney, A.A.; et al. Assessment of recent developmental immunotoxicity studies with bisphenol A in the context of the 2015 EFSA t-TDI. *Reprod. Toxicol.* **2016**, *65*, 448–456. [CrossRef]
11. Lopes-Rocha, L.; Hernandez, C.; Gonçalves, V.; Pinho, T.; Tiritan, M.E. Analytical Methods for Determination of BPA Released from Dental Resin Composites and Related Materials: A Systematic Review. *Crit. Rev. Anal. Chem.* **2024**, *54*, 653–668. [CrossRef]
12. Attik, N.; Hallay, F.; Bois, L.; Brioude, A.; Grosgogeat, B.; Colon, P. Mesoporous silica fillers and resin composition effect on dental composites cytocompatibility. *Dent. Mater.* **2017**, *33*, 166–174. [CrossRef] [PubMed]
13. Yu, B.; Liu, D.; Liu, F.; He, J. Preparation and Characterization of Light-Cured Dental Resin without Methacrylate Monomers Derived from Bisphenol A. *Adv. Polym. Technol.* **2014**, *33*, 21417. [CrossRef]
14. Luo, S.; Zhu, W.; Liu, F.; He, J. Preparation of a Bis-GMA-Free Dental Resin System with Synthesized Fluorinated Dimethacrylate Monomers. *Int. J. Mol. Sci.* **2016**, *17*, 2014. [CrossRef] [PubMed]
15. Fugolin, A.P.; de Paula, A.B.; Dobson, A.; Huynh, V.; Consani, R.; Ferracane, J.L.; Pfeifer, C.S. Alternative monomer for BisGMA-free resin composites formulations. *Dent. Mater.* **2020**, *36*, 884–892. [CrossRef] [PubMed]
16. Hassan, R.; Khan, M.U.A.; Abdullah, A.M.; Razak, S.I.A. A Review on Current Trends of Polymers in Orthodontics: BPA-Free and Smart Materials. *Polymers* **2021**, *13*, 1409. [CrossRef]
17. Sun, Y.; Zhou, Z.; Jiang, H.; Duan, Y.; Li, J.; Liu, X.; Hong, L.; Zhao, C. Preparation and evaluation of novel bio-based Bis-GMA-free dental composites with low estrogenic activity. *Dent. Mater.* **2022**, *38*, 281–293. [CrossRef]
18. He, J.; Kopperud, H.M. Preparation and characterization of Bis-GMA-free dental composites with dimethacrylate monomer derived from 9,9-Bis[4-(2-hydroxyethoxy)phenyl]fluorene. *Dent. Mater.* **2018**, *34*, 1003–1013. [CrossRef]
19. Cidreira Boaro, L.C.; Pereira Lopes, D.; de Souza, A.S.C.; Lie Nakano, E.; Ayala Perez, M.D.; Pfeifer, C.S.; Gonçalves, F. Clinical performance and chemical-physical properties of bulk fill composites resin—A systematic review and meta-analysis. *Dent. Mater.* **2019**, *35*, 249–264. [CrossRef]
20. Ludovichetti, F.S.; Lucchi, P.; Zambon, G.; Pezzato, L.; Bertolini, R.; Zerman, N.; Stellini, E.; Mazzoleni, S. Depth of Cure, Hardness, Roughness and Filler Dimension of Bulk-Fill Flowable, Conventional Flowable and High-Strength Universal Injectable Composites: An In Vitro Study. *Nanomaterials* **2022**, *12*, 1951. [CrossRef]
21. Hatipoğlu, Ö.; Turumtay, E.A.; Saygın, A.G.; Hatipoğlu, F.P. Evaluation of Color Stability of Experimental Dental Composite Resins Prepared from Bis-EFMA, A Novel Monomer System. *J. Photopolym. Sci. Technol.* **2021**, *34*, 297–305. [CrossRef]
22. Hatipoğlu, Ö.; Turumtay, E.A.; Saygın, A.G. Evaluation of monomer elution, microhardness, and roughness of experimental dental composite resins prepared from Bis-EFMA, a novel monomer system. *Polym. Compos.* **2022**, *43*, 584–592. [CrossRef]
23. Zhang, X.; Ma, X.; Liao, M.; Liu, F.; Wei, Q.; Shi, Z.; Mai, S.; He, J. Properties of Bis-GMA free bulk-filled resin composite based on high refractive index monomer Bis-EFMA. *J. Mech. Behav. Biomed. Mater.* **2022**, *134*, 105372. [CrossRef] [PubMed]
24. Ma, X.; Zhang, X.; Huang, X.; Liu, F.; He, J.; Mai, S. Low shrinkage bulk-filled dental resin composites with non-estrogenic dimethacrylate. *Biomater. Sci.* **2023**, *11*, 3669–3682. [CrossRef] [PubMed]
25. Ma, X.; Zhang, X.; Huang, X.; Liu, F.; He, J.; Mai, S. Performance of low shrinkage Bis-EFMA based bulk-fill dental resin composites. *Dent. Mater.* **2024**, *40*, 1378–1389. [CrossRef]
26. *ISO 4049-2019*; Dentistry—Polymer-Based Restorative Materials. International Organization for Standardization: Geneva, Switzerland, 2019.
27. Bucuta, S.; Ilie, N. Light transmittance and micro-mechanical properties of bulk fill vs. conventional resin based composites. *Clin. Oral Investig.* **2014**, *18*, 1991–2000. [CrossRef]
28. Wang, L.; Liu, Y.; Si, W.; Feng, H.; Tao, Y.; Ma, Z. Friction and wear behaviors of dental ceramics against natural tooth enamel. *J. Eur. Ceram. Soc.* **2012**, *32*, 2599–2606. [CrossRef]
29. *ISO 10993-5:2009*; Biological Evaluation of Medical Devices—Part 5: Tests for In Vitro Cytotoxicity. International Organization for Standardization: Geneva, Switzerland, 2009.

30. Palin, W.M.; Leprince, J.G.; Hadis, M.A. Shining a light on high volume photocurable materials. *Dent. Mater.* **2018**, *34*, 695–710. [CrossRef]
31. Moore, B.K.; Platt, J.A.; Borges, G.; Chu, T.-M.G.; Katsilieri, I. Depth of Cure of Dental Resin Composites: ISO 4049 Depth and Microhardness of Types of Materials and Shades. *Oper. Dent.* **2008**, *33*, 408–412. [CrossRef]
32. Paolone, G.; Baldani, S.; De Masi, N.; Mandurino, M.; Collivasone, G.; Scotti, N.; Gherlone, E.; Cantatore, G. Translucency of bulk-fill composite materials: A systematic review. *J. Esthet. Restor. Dent.* **2024**, *36*, 995–1009. [CrossRef]
33. Lee, Y.-K. Influence of filler on the difference between the transmitted and reflected colors of experimental resin composites. *Dent. Mater.* **2008**, *24*, 1243–1247. [CrossRef]
34. Flury, S.; Hayoz, S.; Peutzfeldt, A.; Hüsler, J.; Lussi, A. Depth of cure of resin composites: Is the ISO 4049 method suitable for bulk fill materials? *Dent. Mater.* **2012**, *28*, 521–528. [CrossRef] [PubMed]
35. Colombo, M.; Gallo, S.; Poggio, C.; Ricaldone, V.; Arciola, C.R.; Scribante, A. New Resin-Based Bulk-Fill Composites: In vitro Evaluation of Micro-Hardness and Depth of Cure as Infection Risk Indexes. *Materials* **2020**, *13*, 1308. [CrossRef] [PubMed]
36. Hasanain, F.A.; Nassar, H.M.; Ajaj, R.A. Effect of Light Curing Distance on Microhardness Profiles of Bulk-Fill Resin Composites. *Polymers* **2022**, *14*, 528. [CrossRef] [PubMed]
37. Alrahlah, A.; Silikas, N.; Watts, D.C. Post-cure depth of cure of bulk fill dental resin-composites. *Dent. Mater.* **2014**, *30*, 149–154. [CrossRef]
38. Carrillo-Marcos, A.; Salazar-Correa, G.; Castro-Ramirez, L.; Ladera-Castañeda, M.; López-Gurreonero, C.; Cachay-Criado, H.; Aliaga-Mariñas, A.; Cornejo-Pinto, A.; Cervantes-Ganoza, L.; Cayo-Rojas, C.F. The Microhardness and Surface Roughness Assessment of Bulk-Fill Resin Composites Treated with and without the Application of an Oxygen-Inhibited Layer and a Polishing System: An In Vitro Study. *Polymers* **2022**, *14*, 3053. [CrossRef]
39. Price RB, T.; Felix, C.A.; Andreou, P. Effects of resin composite composition and irradiation distance on the performance of curing lights. *Biomaterials* **2004**, *25*, 4465–4477. [CrossRef]
40. Yılmaz Atalı, P.; Doğu Kaya, B.; Manav Özen, A.; Tarçın, B.; Şenol, A.A.; Tüter Bayraktar, E.; Korkut, B.; Bilgin Göçmen, G.; Tağtekin, D.; Türkmen, C. Assessment of micro-hardness, degree of conversion, and flexural strength for single-shade universal resin composites. *Polymers* **2022**, *14*, 4987. [CrossRef]
41. El-Safty, S.; Akhtar, R.; Silikas, N.; Watts, D. Nanomechanical properties of dental resin-composites. *Dent. Mater.* **2012**, *28*, 1292–1300. [CrossRef]
42. Jun, S.K.; Kim, D.A.; Goo, H.J.; Lee, H.H. Investigation of the correlation between the different mechanical properties of resin composites. *Dent. Mater. J.* **2013**, *32*, 48–57. [CrossRef]
43. Lempel, E.; Czibulya, Z.; Kovács, B.; Szalma, J.; Tóth, Á; Kunsági-Máté, S.; Varga, Z.; Böddi, K. Degree of Conversion and BisGMA, TEGDMA, UDMA Elution from Flowable Bulk Fill Composites. *Int. J. Mol. Sci.* **2016**, *17*, 732. [CrossRef]
44. Amirouche-Korichi, A.; Mouzali, M.; Watts, D.C. Effects of monomer ratios and highly radiopaque fillers on degree of conversion and shrinkage-strain of dental resin composites. *Dent. Mater.* **2009**, *25*, 1411–1418. [CrossRef] [PubMed]
45. Stansbury, J.W. Dimethacrylate network formation and polymer property evolution as determined by the selection of monomers and curing conditions. *Dent. Mater.* **2012**, *28*, 13–22. [CrossRef] [PubMed]
46. Salem, H.; Hefnawy, S.; Nagi, S. Degree of conversion and polymerization shrinkage of low shrinkage bulk-fill resin composites. *Contemp. Clin. Dent.* **2019**, *10*, 465. [CrossRef]
47. Karabela, M.M.; Sideridou, I.D. Synthesis and study of properties of dental resin composites with different nanosilica particles size. *Dent. Mater.* **2011**, *27*, 825–835. [CrossRef]
48. Paolone, G.; Mandurino, M.; Scotti, N.; Cantatore, G.; Blatz, M.B. Color stability of bulk-fill compared to conventional resin-based composites: A scoping review. *J. Esthet. Restor. Dent.* **2023**, *35*, 657–676. [CrossRef] [PubMed]
49. Alshali, R.Z.; Salim, N.A.; Satterthwaite, J.D.; Silikas, N. Long-term sorption and solubility of bulk-fill and conventional resin-composites in water and artificial saliva. *J. Dent.* **2015**, *43*, 1511–1518. [CrossRef]
50. Marovic, D.; Par, M.; Macan, M.; Klarić, N.; Plazonić, I.; Tarle, Z. Aging-Dependent Changes in Mechanical Properties of the New Generation of Bulk-Fill Composites. *Materials* **2022**, *15*, 902. [CrossRef]
51. Althahban, S.; Alomari, A.S.; El-Din MSallam, H.; Jazaa, Y. An investigation of wear, mechanical, and water sorption/solubility behaviors of a commercial restorative composite containing nano-additives. *J. Mater. Res. Technol.* **2023**, *23*, 491–502. [CrossRef]
52. Ferracane, J.L. Placing Dental Composites—A Stressful Experience. *Oper. Dent.* **2008**, *33*, 247–257. [CrossRef]
53. Sampaio, C.S.; Arias, J.F.; Atria, P.J.; Cáceres, E.; Díaz, C.P.; Freitas, A.Z.; Hirata, R. Volumetric polymerization shrinkage and its comparison to internal adaptation in bulk fill and conventional composites: A μCT and OCT in vitro analysis. *Dent. Mater.* **2019**, *35*, 1568–1575. [CrossRef]
54. Guan, X.; Zhu, T.; Zhang, D. Development in polymerization shrinkage control of dental light-cured resin composites: A literature review. *J. Adhes. Sci. Technol.* **2023**, *37*, 602–623. [CrossRef]
55. Par, M.; Marovic, D.; Attin, T.; Tarle, Z.; Tauböck, T.T. Effect of rapid high-intensity light-curing on polymerization shrinkage properties of conventional and bulk-fill composites. *J. Dent.* **2020**, *101*, 103448. [CrossRef] [PubMed]
56. Tauböck, T.T.; Jäger, F.; Attin, T. Polymerization shrinkage and shrinkage force kinetics of high- and low-viscosity dimethacrylate- and ormocer-based bulk-fill resin composites. *Odontology* **2019**, *107*, 103–110. [CrossRef] [PubMed]
57. Algamaiah, H.; Silikas, N.; Watts, D.C. Polymerization shrinkage and shrinkage stress development in ultra-rapid photo-polymerized bulk fill resin composites. *Dent. Mater.* **2021**, *37*, 559–567. [CrossRef] [PubMed]

58. Rizzante, F.A.P.; Mondelli, R.F.L.; Furuse, A.Y.; Borges, A.F.S.; Mendonça, G.; Ishikiriama, S.K. Shrinkage stress and elastic modulus assessment of bulk-fill composites. *J. Appl. Oral Sci.* **2019**, *27*, e20180132. [CrossRef] [PubMed]
59. Yu, P.; Xu, Y.-X.; Liu, Y.-S. Polymerization shrinkage and shrinkage stress of bulk-fill and non-bulk-fill resin-based composites. *J. Dent. Sci.* **2022**, *17*, 1212–1216. [CrossRef]
60. Gonçalves, F.; Pfeifer, C.; Ferracane, J.; Braga, R. Contraction Stress Determinants in Dimethacrylate Composites. *J. Dent. Res.* **2008**, *87*, 367–371. [CrossRef]
61. Eweis, A.; Yap, A.; Yahya, N. Comparison of Flexural Properties of Bulk-fill Restorative/Flowable Composites and Their Conventional Counterparts. *Oper. Dent.* **2020**, *45*, 41–51. [CrossRef]
62. Dahri, W.M.; Kumar, N.; Altaf, N.; Mughal, W.; Zafar, M.S. Mechanical and Biomimetic Characteristics of Bulk-Fill Resin Dental Composites Following Exposure in a Simulated Acidic Oral Environment. *Biomimetics* **2023**, *8*, 19. [CrossRef]
63. Ilie, N.; Moldovan, M.; Ionescu, A.C. Microstructure and Mechanical Behavior of Modern Universal-Chromatic and Bulk-Fill Resin-Based Composites Developed to Simplify Dental Restorative Procedures. *J. Funct. Biomater.* **2022**, *13*, 178. [CrossRef]
64. Shah, P.K.; Stansbury, J.W. Role of filler and functional group conversion in the evolution of properties in polymeric dental restoratives. *Dent. Mater.* **2014**, *30*, 586–593. [CrossRef] [PubMed]
65. Goracci, C.; Cadenaro, M.; Fontanive, L.; Giangrosso, G.; Juloski, J.; Vichi, A.; Ferrari, M. Polymerization efficiency and flexural strength of low-stress restorative composites. *Dent. Mater.* **2014**, *30*, 688–694. [CrossRef] [PubMed]
66. Finan, L.; Palin, W.M.; Moskwa, N.; McGinley, E.L.; Fleming, G.J. The influence of irradiation potential on the degree of conversion and mechanical properties of two bulk-fill flowable RBC base materials. *Dent. Mater.* **2013**, *29*, 906–912. [CrossRef]
67. Fronza, B.; Ayres, A.; Pacheco, R.; Rueggeberg, F.; Dias, C.; Giannini, M. Characterization of inorganic filler content, mechanical properties, and light transmission of Bulk-fill resin composites. *Oper. Dent.* **2017**, *42*, 445–455. [CrossRef]
68. Szczesio-Wlodarczyk, A.; Sokolowski, J.; Kleczewska, J.; Bociong, K. Ageing of Dental Composites Based on Methacrylate Resins—A Critical Review of the Causes and Method of Assessment. *Polymers* **2020**, *12*, 882. [CrossRef]
69. Ferracane, J.L.; Berge, H.X.; Condon, J.R. In vitro aging of dental composites in water—Effect of degree of conversion, filler volume, and filler/matrix coupling. *J. Biomed. Mater. Res.* **1998**, *42*, 465–472. [CrossRef]
70. Osiewicz, M.A.; Werner, A.; Roeters, F.J.; Kleverlaan, C.J. Wear of bulk-fill resin composites. *Dent. Mater.* **2022**, *38*, 549–553. [CrossRef]
71. Shimokawa, C.; Giannini, M.; André, C.; Sahadi, B.; Faraoni, J.; Palma-Dibb, R.; Soares, C.; Price, R. In Vitro Evaluation of Surface Properties and Wear Resistance of Conventional and Bulk-fill Resin-based Composites after Brushing with a Dentifrice. *Oper. Dent.* **2019**, *44*, 637–647. [CrossRef] [PubMed]
72. Hu, X.; Marquis, P.M.; Shortall, A.C. Influence of filler loading on the two-body wear of a dental composite. *J. Oral Rehabil.* **2003**, *30*, 729–737. [CrossRef]
73. Matsuura, T.; Komatsu, K.; Choi, K.; Suzumura, T.; Cheng, J.; Chang, T.-L.; Chao, D.; Ogawa, T. Conditional Mitigation of Dental-Composite Material-Induced Cytotoxicity by Increasing the Cure Time. *J. Funct. Biomater.* **2023**, *14*, 119. [CrossRef]
74. Lim, S.M.; Yap, A.; Loo, C.; Ng, J.; Goh, C.Y.; Hong, C.; Toh, W.S. Comparison of cytotoxicity test models for evaluating resin-based composites. *Hum. Exp. Toxicol.* **2017**, *36*, 339–348. [CrossRef] [PubMed]
75. Wiertelak-Makała, K.; Szymczak-Pajor, I.; Bociong, K.; Śliwińska, A. Considerations about Cytotoxicity of Resin-Based Composite Dental Materials: A Systematic Review. *Int. J. Mol. Sci.* **2024**, *25*, 152. [CrossRef] [PubMed]
76. Demïrel, G.; Gür, G.; Demïrsoy, F.F.; Altuntaş, E.G.; Yener-Ilce, B.; Kiliçarslan, M.A. Cytotoxic effects of contemporary bulk-fill dental composites: A real-time cell analysis. *Dent. Mater. J.* **2020**, *39*, 101–110. [CrossRef] [PubMed]
77. Shajii, L.; Santerre, J.P. Effect of filler content on the profile of released biodegradation products in micro-filled Bis-GMA/TEGDMA dental composite resins. *Biomaterials* **1999**, *20*, 1897–1908. [CrossRef]

materials

MDPI

Article

Effect of a 4 mm vs. a 6 mm Diameter Mold on the Depth of Cure of 6 Bulk-Fill Resin-Based Composites

Anubhav Gulati, Alexandre P. Gareau and Richard B. Price *

Department of Dental Clinical Sciences, Faculty of Dentistry, Dalhousie University, Halifax, NS B3H 4R2, Canada; an623775@dal.ca (A.G.); alex.gareau@dal.ca (A.P.G.)

* Correspondence: rbprice@dal.ca; Tel.: +1-902-494-1912

Abstract: Dental researchers and manufacturers use the ISO 4049 standard to determine the depth of cure (DoC) of resin-based composites (RBCs). This standard uses a 4 mm diameter stainless-steel mold and subsequently divides the length of the remaining hard RBC by 2. However, the DoC values obtained using this mold have been challenged. Six bulk-fill RBCs (Tetric plus Fill, Tetric plus Flow, Tetric PowerFill, Tetric PowerFlow, Filtek One, and Aura Bulk Fill) were used to investigate the limitations of the 4 mm diameter mold used in the ISO 4049 standard when compared to a 6 mm diameter metal mold that represented the dimensions of a large cavity in a tooth. Two distinct light curing units were used. One light (Elipar S10) emitted a single peak wavelength of light, while the other (Bluephase G4) was a broad-spectrum, multiple-peak curing light. After 10 s of photocuring, the uncured RBC was immediately removed using acetone. The maximum length of the hard RBC remaining was measured and divided by two so that the effect of these two mold diameters on the DoC results could be compared. The DoC of all six RBCs tested was consistently greater in the 6 mm diameter mold ($p < 0.0001$). Sectioning revealed that the solvent-dissolved specimens had a clear internal boundary between the apparently well-cured RBC and a peripheral, solvent-resistant, "frosty" region. Using a 4 mm diameter stainless-steel mold resulted in a reduced depth of cure values compared to those obtained when the 6 mm diameter mold was used. The use of a broad-spectrum, multiple-peak LED curing light proved unnecessary for photocuring the six RBCs used in this study.

Keywords: resin-based composite; depth of cure; effect of mold diameter; ISO 4049 standard

1. Introduction

Following international agreements to reduce the use of amalgam [1] and regulatory changes in the European Union banning the use of amalgam [2], photopolymerized resin-based composites (RBCs) have become the predominant direct restorative material. Consequently, significant research has focused on determining the polymerization metrics and how they relate to the light curing unit (LCU), the RBC, and the dimensions of the restoration. The polymerization of RBCs is frequently determined by measuring the depth of cure (DoC) according to the international ISO 4049 standard [3,4], by mechanical property testing, or by measuring the degree of conversion (DC) [4,5], where the DC refers to the percentage of monomer molecules that have been successfully converted into polymer chains during curing [5]. Many in vitro studies have shown that undercuring will produce a weaker RBC that is more prone to fracture, has a lower bond strength to the tooth, releases more chemical leachates into the mouth, and has more microleakage [6–10]. One in vivo study [11] placed RBC restorations in denture teeth and reported increased wear when these RBCs received inadequate light exposure.

1.1. Tests Measuring Depth of Cure (DoC)

In the ISO 4049 standard [3] Depth of Cure test, the RBC specimen is made in a 4 mm diameter stainless-steel mold over white filter paper. The specimen is removed immediately after light exposure, and the uncured RBC is manually scraped away using a plastic spatula [3]. The maximum length of the remaining hard, cured RBC cylinder is then measured. This maximum length is divided by two and reported as the "depth of cure" for that RBC and exposure time. This ISO standard only requires that two test specimens be made.

1.2. Limitations of the ISO 4049 Test

While the ISO 4049 DoC test [3] offers simplicity and ease of implementation, it makes no claims regarding correlation with the degree of conversion or the clinical performance of the RBC. In practice, cavities vary considerably in configuration and depth; few match the 4 mm diameter used in the ISO 4049 test, and none are surrounded by metal. The operator technique [12]; the type of mold material, backing, and mold diameter [13–18]; and the beam profile [19,20] are known to all affect the DoC values obtained using the ISO 4049 standard. The use of a 6 mm diameter metal mold, compared to a 4 mm diameter mold, has been reported to increase the DoC by between 6% and 8% [16]. Others have used the 6 mm diameter mold [21,22] to determine the DoC. In 2019, Erickson et al. [18] showed that RBCs that were photo-cured in a 4 mm diameter mold made from a tooth had DoCs that were significantly greater (28–35%) than those obtained from the 4 mm diameter stainless-steel mold. They reported that the ISO 4049 standard test using a 4 mm diameter metal mold was a conservative method for determining the DoC in a tooth. In addition, the DoC test described in the ISO 4049 standard only measures the maximum length of RBC remaining. Since the RBC remaining has been reported [15,18,21,23] to have a dome or "bullet-shape" appearance, this maximum length does not reflect the DoC in a tooth cavity. Also, manually removing the uncured RBC can be very subjective depending on the operator's technique, the stiffness or sharpness of the plastic spatula, or the consistency of the RBC [12]. Instead, it would be ideal to remove uncured dental resin reproducibly using a "no-touch" approach where a solvent such as ethanol, butanone, or acetone [4,12,21–28] is used to remove the uncured resin. Using such a "no-touch" solvent dissolution technique may prevent the DoC value from being over or under-estimated.

1.3. Clinical Relevance of a 4 mm Diameter Metal Mold to Test DoC of Bulk-Fill RBCs

Some modern direct restoratives are designed for bulk photocuring in increments that are 4 to 5 mm thick. When considering typical cavity dimensions—with mandibular premolars averaging 7.0 mm in mesio-distal width, 7.5 mm in bucco-lingual dimension coronally, and 5.0 mm by 6.5 mm at the cervical margin [29]—testing the polymerization of a small 4 mm diameter specimen provides minimal insight into the ability of the LCU to simultaneously polymerize the mesial and distal boxes of a bulk-filled MOD restoration in a premolar tooth, let alone a larger molar tooth. The test results may be further complicated by a non-uniform distribution of light coming from the light tip of the LCU [19–21,23,28]. Areas of high irradiance will produce inconsistent polymerization patterns and artificially enhanced readings directly beneath the irradiance peaks, the "hot spots" of high irradiance [19–21,28]. It is well reported that many LCUs have these "hot spots" of high irradiance, often at the center of the light tip [19–21,28,30,31] and even have an uneven emission spectrum across the light tip [21,31]. Consequently, if a 4 mm diameter mold is positioned under an area of high local irradiance, or a different range of wavelengths, then the results produced may not represent the DoC that would be achieved if the RBC is positioned under a different region of the light tip [19–21,28].

1.4. Research Objectives and Hypotheses

Despite substantial evidence that mold dimensions and materials affect the DoC [13–18,20,21], the ISO 4049 standard [3] continues to use 4 mm diameter stainless-steel molds to test the DoC of all photocured RBCs. Therefore, this study examined the effect of using this 4 mm diameter mold compared to a 6 mm diameter mold [15,16,21,22,32] on the DoC measurements for six contemporary bulk-fill RBCs. Additionally, since previous research suggests multi-wavelength sources may not always be necessary [33–35], the performance of a single-peak-wavelength LCU was compared to a multiple-wavelength LCU.

The hypotheses tested were as follows:

(1) Increasing the mold diameter from 4 to 6 mm will not significantly affect the DoC measurements of the six RBCs tested.
(2) No significant difference will exist between DoC values obtained using single-wavelength or multi-wavelength light sources.

2. Materials and Methods

The DoC was measured for six different bulk-fill RBCs: Tetric plus Fill, Tetric plus Flow, Tetric PowerFill, Tetric PowerFlow, Filtek One, and Aura Bulk Fill (Table 1). The samples of each RBC light were photo-cured using a Bluephase G4 (SN1400002115, Ivoclar Vivadent, Schaan, Liechtenstein) or the Elipar S10 (1016016495, 3 M, St. Paul, MN, USA) light-emitting diode (LED) light. The Bluephase G4 light is a multiple-peak LCU manufactured by the makers of Tetric plus Fill, Tetric plus Flow, Tetric PowerFill, and Tetric PowerFlow. In contrast, the Elipar S10 light is a single-wavelength LED light manufactured by the same company that produces Filtek One.

Table 1. Manufacturers' location, lot numbers, shades, initiators, and the minimum irradiance values recommended by the manufacturers [36–38] of the bulk-fill RBCs used in the study.

RBC	Manufacturer	Lot Number	Shade	Initiator	Minimum Irradiance and Recommended Wavelength Range
Tetric plus Fill	Ivoclar Vivadent, Schaan, Liechtenstein	YM0206	A3	Camphorquinone plus Ivocerin	900–1400 mW/cm^2 for 10 s in the 400–500 nm range
Tetric plus Flow	Ivoclar Vivadent, Schaan, Liechtenstein	YM0210	A3	Camphorquinone plus Ivocerin	900–1400 mW/cm^2 for 10 s in the 400–500 nm range
Tetric PowerFill	Ivoclar Vivadent, Schaan, Liechtenstein	Z06955	IVA	Camphorquinone plus Ivocerin	900–1400 mW/cm^2 for 10 s in the 400–500 nm range
Tetric PowerFlow	Ivoclar Vivadent, Schaan, Liechtenstein	Z06P1N	IVA	Camphorquinone plus Ivocerin	900–1400 mW/cm^2 for 10 s in the 400–500 nm range
Filtek One	3 M, St. Paul, MN, USA	4867A3	A3	Camphorquinone	1000–2000 mW/cm^2 for 20 s in the 400–500 nm range
Aura Bulk Fill	SDI, Bayswater, Victoria, Australia	1222869	Universal	Camphorquinone	High-power LED curing light for 20 s in the 460–480 nm range

2.1. LCU Radiant Power and Beam Profile

The radiant powers from the Bluephase G4 and the Elipar S10 delivered to the 4 and the 6 mm diameter test specimens were recorded five times using a 6 inch integrating sphere (Labsphere, North Sutton, NH, USA) connected to a fiber optic spectrometer (USB 4000, Ocean Optics, Dunedin, FL, USA). The measurement system was calibrated with a traceable reference standard light before testing commenced. The light output from each LCU was measured through a 4 mm or a 6 mm diameter aperture into the sphere that matched the diameter of the 4 mm and the 6 mm diameter molds used for the DoC tests. The LCU tips were centered over this aperture at 0 mm from the entrance into the integrating sphere. The irradiance distribution across the light guide tip end was then characterized using a previously described laser beam profiler technique [20] to produce color-scaled images of the irradiance distribution and radiant exposure across the end of the light guide. The laser beam analyzer camera (Model SP620U, Ophir-Spiricon, Logan, UT, USA) was focused onto the surface of a 60° holographic diffuser target (54-505; Edmund Optics, Barrington, NJ, USA). Two blue bandpass filters (34-434; Edmund Optics) and one spectrally flat reflective neutral density filter (Edmund Optics) were used to flatten the spectral response of the camera, ensuring that the violet and blue wavelengths of light were recorded equally. The beam profile images were recorded using software (BeamGage Professional version 6.21.1, Ophir-Spiricon). The BeamGage software added a 4 mm or a 6 mm diameter circle defining the beam image, and the mean radiant power values (mW) previously obtained using the integrating sphere were inserted into the BeamGage software to produce color-coded irradiance (mW/cm^2) value images within the 4 mm or 6 mm diameter circles. These values were then multiplied by the exposure time (10 s) to produce calibrated radiant exposure images.

2.2. Depth of Cure (DoC) of RBCs

The uncured resin-based composites (RBCs) were placed into stainless-steel molds with either 4 mm or 6 mm diameter internal openings positioned over a white filter paper background, following the ISO 4049 standard [3]. These metal molds were 10 mm deep, and the 6 mm diameter openings represented a more clinically relevant, larger-diameter restoration than the 4 mm diameter molds. A polyester strip was positioned over each surface of the RBC before it was light-cured for 10 s, with the tip end of the LCU placed directly against the polyester surface and centered above the mold opening. The LCUs were firmly secured in position throughout the experiment, and all specimens were prepared in a random order at room temperature (approximately 22 °C), maintaining the same LCU/tip/mold orientation.

A total of 120 specimens were created (2 diameters × 6 RBCs × 5 replications × 2 LCUs). Immediately following light exposure, the polyester strips were removed, the molds were opened, and the RBC was removed. The soft, uncured RBC was left intact and not scraped away. Instead, the RBC specimen was promptly submerged in an organic solvent (Acetone, Sigma Aldrich, St. Louis, MO, USA) for 15 min at 22 °C. After removing the RBC specimens from the solvent, they were air-dried. A trained operator measured the maximum length of the specimens using digital calipers (Mitutoyo, Canada Inc., Mississauga, ON, Canada). Following the ISO 4049 standard [3], these values were divided by 2 to report the DoC in mm for each RBC. Representative specimens were cut in half longitudinally, and standardized digital photographs were taken to determine the shape of the specimens and to see if a previously documented [21,25] "frosty" layer was present at the bottom of the RBCs.

2.3. Statistics

The DoC results for each RBC were normally distributed. Analyses of Variance (ANOVAs) were then used to determine the impact of the RBC, LCU, and mold diameter on the length of the remaining hard RBC (StatView for Windows v.5.0; SAS Institute, Cary, NC, USA). The effects of mold diameter and the use of Bluephase G4 vs. Elipar S10 for 10 s were compared using Tukey–Kramer multiple comparison tests. All tests used a significance level of $\alpha = 0.05$. The RBCs were not compared because the same exposure time (10 s) was used for all the RBCs, and this time was not always the manufacturer's recommended exposure time.

3. Results

3.1. Radiant Power and Beam Profile

Figures 1 and 2 illustrate the differences in the spectral radiant powers and irradiance distributions delivered to the top surface of the 4 and 6 mm diameter molds from the two LCUs. As expected, Elipar S10 was a single-peak LCU delivering only blue light. The Elipar S10 had a region of high irradiance (mW/cm^2) at the center that delivered a greater radiant exposure (J/cm^2) to the center of the RBC in the mold (Figure 2). The Bluephase G4 was a multiple-peak LCU that delivered both violet and blue light, and it had a more uniform irradiance and radiant exposure beam profile.

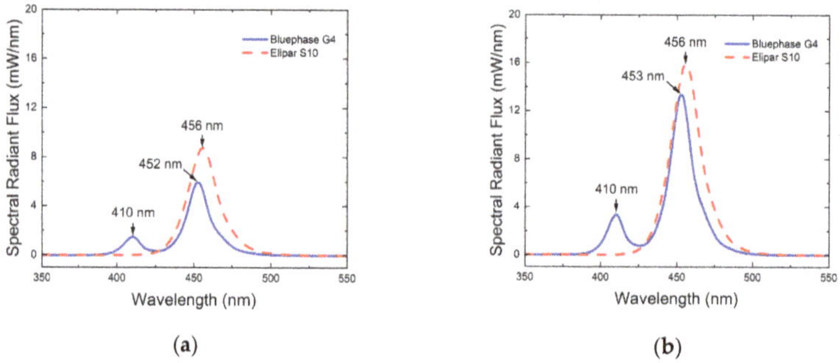

Figure 1. Light received by the 4 mm (**a**) and 6 mm (**b**) diameter specimens. Note the different emission spectra and the different spectral radiant flux delivered to the 4 mm diameter and the 6 mm diameter molds.

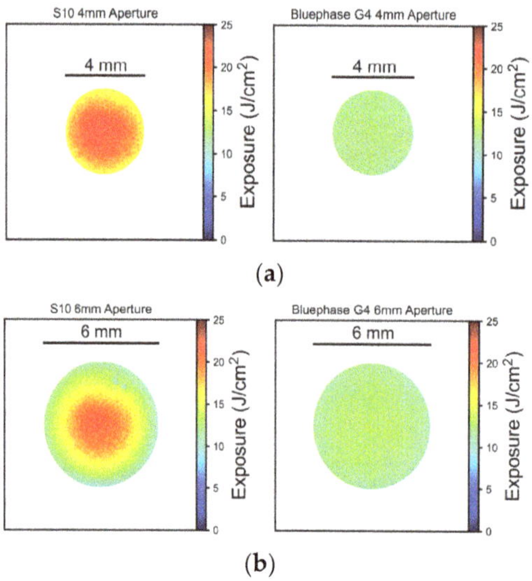

Figure 2. Beam profiles of the radiant exposure (J/cm^2) received by the 4 mm (**a**) and 6 mm (**b**) diameter specimens from the S10 and the G4 lights in 10 s. Note the inhomogeneous distribution of light and energy from the S10 curing light with a "hot spot" at the center of the light tip.

When measured through the 4 mm diameter aperture into the integrating sphere, the radiant power from the Bluephase G4 LCU was 152 mW, while the Elipar S10's was

55% greater at 236 mW. When measured through the 6 mm diameter aperture, the radiant power from the Bluephase G4 LCU was 345 mW, but the Elipar S10's was only 24% greater at 427 mW. Thus, in 10 s, Bluephase G4 delivered 3.45 J, while Elipar S10 delivered 4.27 J to the 6 mm diameter specimens. However, the 4 mm diameter specimens only received 1.52 J from Bluephase G4 and 2.36 J from Elipar S10 in 10 s.

3.2. Remaining Cured Composite Remnant Thickness and Depth of Cure (DoC)

Depending on the test condition, after 10 s of light exposure, the mean length of hard RBC remaining ranged from 5.2 mm to 10.0 mm, or from 2.6 mm to 5 mm when divided by 2 (Table 2). See also Supplemental Figure S1 illustrating the differences in the DoC.

Table 2. Mean length (mm) divided by 2 of the hard resin-based composite (RBC) remaining, depending on the mold diameter and LCU used. Shaded cells represent DoC values that were greater than 4 mm. The increase (%) when the 6 mm diameter mold was used compared to the 4 mm diameter mold is also reported.

RBC, Mold Diameter and LCU	Length (mm)	S.D.	Increase (%) Using the 6 mm Diameter Mold
PowerFlow, 6 mm, S10	5	0.01	19.0%
PowerFlow, 6 mm, G4	4.9	0.02	22.5%
Filtek One, 6 mm, S10	4.2	0.09	10.5%
PowerFlow, 4 mm, S10	4.2	0.08	
PowerFill, 6 mm, S10	4.1	0.09	17.1%
Tetric plus Flow, 6 mm, S10	4.1	0.04	13.9%
PowerFlow, 4 mm, G4	4	0.04	
Filtek One, 4 mm, S10	3.8	0.03	
PowerFill, 6 mm, G4	3.8	0.08	15.2%
Tetric plus Fill, 6 mm, S10	3.8	0.08	11.8%
Tetric plus Flow, 6 mm, G4	3.8	0.05	11.8%
Filtek One, 6 mm, G4	3.7	0.04	10.8%
Tetric plus Fill, 6 mm, G4	3.6	0.13	12.5%
Tetric plus Flow, 4 mm, S10	3.6	0.12	
PowerFill, 4 mm, S10	3.5	0.12	
Tetric plus Fill, 4 mm, S10	3.4	0.11	
Tetric plus Flow, 4 mm, G4	3.4	0.03	
Filtek One, 4 mm, G4	3.3	0.04	
PowerFill, 4 mm, G4	3.3	0.05	
Tetric plus Fill, 4 mm, G4	3.2	0.06	
AuraBulk, 6 mm, S10	3.1	0.07	14.8%
AuraBulk, 6 mm, G4	2.9	0.07	11.5%
AuraBulk, 4 mm, S10	2.7	0.08	
AuraBulk, 4 mm, G4	2.6	0.04	

The ANOVA results showed that all the factors (RBC, mold diameter, and LCU) had a significant effect on the DoC. The mold diameter ($p < 0.0001$, F = 1407.90, the highest F-value) had the greatest effect. The choice of RBC also had a substantial impact ($p < 0.0001$, F = 1070.28), but this was less than the effect of the mold diameter. For all six RBCs, the 6 mm diameter mold always produced a greater depth of cure compared to the 4 mm diameter mold ($p < 0.0001$). The Tetric PowerFlow, photo-cured using the single-peak S10 light source in the 6 mm diameter mold, produced the greatest DoC of 5.0 mm.

There was a significant interaction effect between the RBC and mold diameter ($p < 0.0001$, F = 32.40). Although this interaction between the RBC and diameter was significant, Table 3 shows that this effect was weaker and had a much lower F value (F = 32.40) than the main effects of mold diameter (F = 1407.90) or the RBC (F = 1070.28). Thus, the effect of the 4 mm and 6 mm diameter mold on the DoC was not always as strong across the six RBCs. The Tukey–Kramer multiple comparison tests confirmed that there were significant differences between the RBCs and sample conditions. Although Elipar S10 produced a 10.5% to 19.0% increase in the DoC in the 6 mm diameter molds and Bluephase G4 produced a 10.8% to 22.5% increase in the DoC in the 6 mm diameter molds, overall, the Elipar S10 light produced a significantly greater DoC ($p = 0.018$) than Bluephase G4 (Table 2).

Table 3. ANOVA results showing the effects of the resin-based composite (RBC), the mold diameter, and the LCU on the length of hard RBC remaining.

Factor	DF	Sum of Squares	Mean Square	F-Value	*p*-Value	Power
RBC	5	29.35	5.87	1070.28	<0.0001	1.0
Mold Diameter	1	7.72	7.72	1407.90	<0.0001	1.0
LCU	1	1.88	1.88	342.79	<0.0001	1.0
RBC*Mold Diameter	5	0.89	0.18	32.40	<0.0001	1.0
RBC*LCU	5	0.32	0.06	11.67	<0.0001	1.0
Mold Diameter* Light	1	0.00	0.00	0.37	0.55	0.09
RBC*Mold Diameter* LCU	5	0.06	0.01	2.26	0.05	0.71
Residual	96	0.53	0.01			1.0

3.3. *Bottom Surface Topography*

When sectioned longitudinally in half, the remaining hard RBC had an unsymmetrical bottom surface profile (see Figure 3 for the 4 mm diameter specimens and Figure 4 for the 6 mm diameter specimens). The ends of the RBC specimens had a distinct "bullet" shape, and a "frosty" layer of partially solvent-resistant RBC was present at the bottom of all the RBCs.

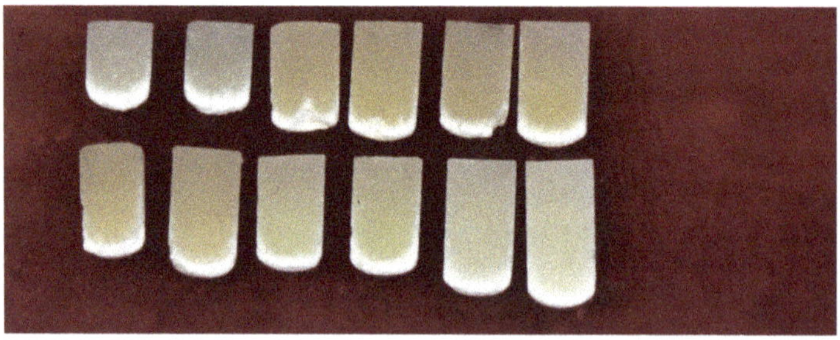

Figure 3. Sectioned 4 mm diameter specimens photocured using the G4 and S10 LCUs showing a cross-section of the remaining hard RBC. Note the "bullet"-shaped appearance and the "frosty" layer in all the images. The RBCs and LCUs used are in the following order from left to right: **TOP ROW:** Aura Bulk Fill G4, Aura Bulk Fill S10; Tetric plus Fill G4, Tetric plus Fill S10; Tetric plus Flow G4, Tetric plus Flow S10. **BOTTOM ROW:** Filtek One G4, Filtek One S10; Tetric PowerFill G4, Tetric PowerFill S10; Tetric PowerFlow G4, Tetric PowerFlow S10.

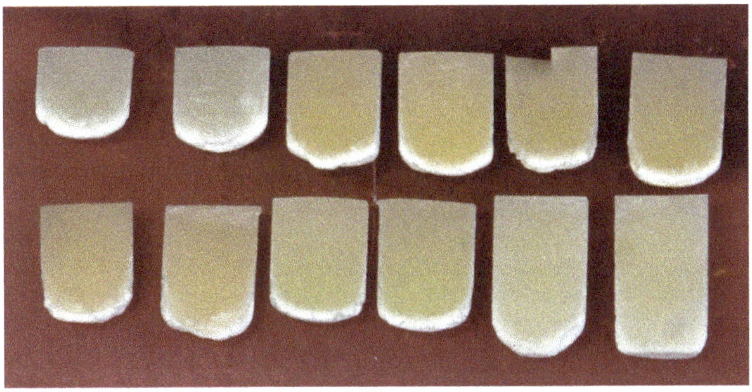

Figure 4. Sectioned 6 mm diameter specimens photocured using the G4 and S10 LCUs showing a cross-section of the remaining hard RBC. Note the "bullet"-shaped appearance and the "frosty" layer in àll the images. The RBCs and LCUs used are in the following order from left to right. **TOP ROW:** Aura Bulk Fill G4, Aura Bulk Fill S10; Tetric plus Fill G4, Tetric plus fill S10; Tetric plus Flow G4, Tetric plus Flow S10. **BOTTOM ROW:** Filtek One G4, Filtek One S10; Tetric PowerFill G4, Tetric PowerFill S10; Tetric PowerFlow G4, Tetric PowerFlow S10.

4. Discussion

This investigation required only one RBC to have a significant difference in the DoC achieved in the 4 mm and 6 mm diameter molds to question the results from the current ISO 4049 standard. Instead, all six RBCs achieved a 10.5 to 22.5% increase in the DoC in the 6 mm diameter molds (Table 2). This was very significantly greater than the DoC results achieved in the 4 mm diameter molds ($p < 0.0001$). Thus, the first research hypothesis was rejected. Furthermore, the Elipar S10 single-peak-wavelength LCU that delivered greater total energy with a "hot spot" of high irradiance at the center (Figure 4) consistently produced greater DoC values ($p = 0.018$) compared to the multiple-peak wavelength LCU that had a more uniform output distribution (Table 2); thus, the second hypothesis that there would be no difference between the LCUs was rejected.

As illustrated in Figures 3 and 4, except for the Tetric PowerFlow that had been exposed to the S10 light for 10 s in the 6 mm diameter mold, the remaining RBCs were all dome-shaped, and a "frosty" layer was present at the bottom (Figure 4). Had the 6 mm diameter metal mold been longer, the DoC of the Tetric PowerFlow would likely have been slightly longer in the 6 mm diameter mold. A similar dome or "bullet-shape" appearance and increased hardness at the center of RBC specimens compared to the outer regions have been reported previously [14,15,17–19,21,23]. Previous studies have also reported that the hardness of the RBC photocured in opaque molds was substantially lower at or near the walls of the mold than at the center and that the depth of cure was also dependent on the diameter of the mold [14,15,18,19,21]. While this may be due to the opaque nature of the mold [14], this effect may also be attributed to the fact that not all surface areas of the specimen received the same radiant exposure from the LCU [19]. This was illustrated in Figure 2, where the S10 light delivered more energy to the RBC at the center of the mold. This inhomogeneous distribution of light across the light tip may be the reason why the "bullet-shaped" curing pattern was observed in the RBCs [23], but since the G4 delivered a homogeneous distribution of light, this "bullet-shaped" curing pattern may also be due to the thermal mass of the stainless-steel mold that reduced the temperature increase in the RBC that was close to the metal walls as it polymerized [23]. This reduced the beneficial effect of the exothermic temperature increases that occurred during polymerization.

The ISO 4049 standard only requires a sample size of 2. The present study used a sample size of 5, and the statistical power values were 1.0, confirming that the sample size and statistical tests were highly effective in detecting differences. As shown in Figures 3 and 4 and Tables 2 and 3, the mold diameter caused a 10.5 to 22.5% increase in the DoC in the 6 mm diameter molds and was the most significant factor that affected the length of the remaining hard RBC ($p < 0.0001$). Despite the large volume increase in the total amount of material used in the 6 mm diameter mold compared to the 4 mm diameter mold (from 125.7 mm^3 to 282.7 mm^3), when the RBCs were exposed using the same 10 s exposure time, the length of the remaining hard RBC remaining always increased as the mold diameter increased from 4 mm to 6 mm. This may be because Bluephase G4 delivered 3.45 J, whereas Elipar S10 delivered 4.27 J to the 6 mm diameter specimens in 10 s. In contrast, the 4 mm diameter specimens only received 1.52 J from Bluephase G4 and 2.36 J from Elipar S10 in 10 s. Thus, although the volume of the 6 mm diameter mold was greater, the greater DoC achieved in the 6 mm diameter mold is likely because the RBC in the 6 mm diameter mold received more energy from both LCUs. The fact that more energy was delivered from the single-peak Elipar S10 light also explains why the Elipar S10 produced a significantly greater DoC ($p = 0.018$) compared to the multi-peak G4. This observation that the Elipar S10 LCU delivered 55% more energy than the Bluephase G4 through the 4 mm aperture, but only 24% more energy through the 6 mm aperture, highlights the irradiance beam's non-uniformity delivered by Elipar S10. This LCU has now been replaced by the Elipar Deep Cure, which has a more uniform beam profile.

This study did not conduct a chemical analysis of the photoinitiators used in the six RBCs tested. However, four of these RBCs, Tetric plus Fill, Tetric plus Flow, Tetric PowerFill G4, and Tetric PowerFlow, are made by Ivoclar. These RBCs use a combination of camphorquinone and Ivocerin [36], while the manufacturers of Aura Bulk Fill and Filtek One state that these RBCs use only camphorquinone [37,38]. Filtek One, Tetric PowerFlow, Tetric PowerFill, and Tetric plus Flow produced test specimens that were at least 4 mm long in the 6 mm diameter mold after a 10 s exposure using the single-peak Elipar S10 light (Table 2). This result confirms other reports that a multiple-wavelength peak LCU is not always required [33–35].

In clinical practice, cavities vary in shape and depth, and multiple variables influence the DoC, including the presence of adjacent walls and the cavity size. While the ISO 4049 standard, which uses a 4 mm diameter mold is a simple screening method, it only measures the maximum length of hard RBC remaining. The resulting depth of cure values are, therefore, highly dependent upon the operator [12], the maximum length measurement, and the beam homogeneity of the LCU. Given the "bullet-shaped" appearance of the RBCs, it is important to report the shape of the hard RBC remaining. Placing the RBC in acetone for 15 min was considered less aggressive than the Acetone Shake Test [12,27], where the RBC is placed in acetone in an amalgamator and vibrated for 15 s. This vibration jostles the RBC and mechanically removes some of the RBC. Instead, this study's 15 min immersion "no-touch" technique removed the uncured RBC without any physical contact. This eliminated the operator's subjective judgment and any inconsistent performance when scraping away the uncured RBC [12,21,22,25,26].

When the solvent-dissolved RBC specimens were sectioned, a clear internal boundary between the RBC that was apparently well-cured, and the peripheral, porous, solvent-resistant polymer could be seen. This region has been previously characterized as "frosty" [21,25]. This "frosty" region followed the contour of the hard bottom surface of the RBC (Figures 3 and 4) and was approximately 1.0 to 1.5 mm wide. Its width appears to be visually similar to the 2.2 mm difference between the length of hard RBC that remains after the soft RBC has been scraped away and the region where clinically relevant differences in the RBC properties have been reported to begin [24]. As illustrated in Figure 3 (the 4 mm diameter specimens) and Figure 4 (the 6 mm diameter specimens), this "frosty" region never penetrated into the first half of the RBC closest to the light. The presence and configuration of this porous region suggest that the method used in the ISO 4049 standard [3] of reporting half the maximum length of the remaining hard RBC as the depth of cure (DoC) may provide inaccurately short DoC values.

Since the manufacturer's recommended exposure times were not always used, the study did not compare the DoC of the RBCs. When using this 10 s exposure, Aura Bulk Fill produced the shortest DoC of 2.6 to 3.1 mm, depending on the mold and LCU used (Table 3). This was likely because Aura Bulk Fill and Filtek One received only half of their recommended exposure times (Table 1). This result supports the conclusions of a previous study [22] that reported the importance of following the instructions for use provided by the manufacturer of the RBC, not those of the manufacturer of the LCU.

While the results obtained using a 4 mm diameter metal mold can provide a standard laboratory test, its relevance in the clinical setting where most cavities are larger than 4 mm in diameter is uncertain [39]. Since the RBCs photocured in the 6 mm diameter mold consistently yielded higher DoC values, this finding supports Erickson et al.'s [18] conclusion that modifications to the current ISO 4049 standard [3] are necessary. While the influences of the mold's thermal mass, volume, and solvent immersion duration have yet to be fully determined, using a 6 mm diameter mold may provide outcomes that are more clinically relevant than the 4 mm diameter mold currently specified in the ISO 4049 standard.

The purpose of this study was to demonstrate and confirm that there were significant differences in the DoC values between the 4 and 6 mm diameter molds. The 6 mm diameter mold has been used previously by others [15,16,21,22] and was chosen to represent a large restoration in a premolar tooth. A wider, e.g., 7 mm diameter mold, would have been wider than the active diameter of some light guides [19,28], and, thus, the RBC in the mold would not have received direct light. Thus, a 6 mm diameter mold appears to be the largest that can be used.

Although this study found that the 6 mm diameter mold always produced a greater depth of cure in the six bulk-fill RBCs tested, not all available RBCs were tested. Additionally, a standard 10 s exposure time was used for all RBCs to minimize the number of variables in the study. This time was shorter than the manufacturer's recommended exposure time for Filtek One and Aura Bulk Fill, which was why the DoC between the RBCs was not compared. Future studies into the DoC of RBCs could use a mold that better simulates a human tooth's shape, thermal properties, and light transmission characteristics. Future studies should develop specific guidelines for identifying the ideal solvent and the optimal duration of solvent exposure. Given the "bullet-shaped" appearance of the RBCs, future studies should also report the shape of the hard RBC remaining. Ongoing microhardness tests and degree of conversion analyses are attempting to identify the nature of the polymerization along the "frosty layer" at the bottom of the solvent-dissolved RBCs.

5. Conclusions

This study showed that

1. The 6 mm diameter metal molds consistently produced greater depth-of-cure results than standard 4 mm diameter configurations specified in the ISO 4049 standard ($p < 0.0001$).
2. The single-peak-wavelength LCU provided equivalent or superior performance compared to the multiple-peak-wavelength LCU tested in this study.

3. The RBC polymerized in the metal molds consistently exhibited a dome-shaped morphology with a greater DoC at the center compared to the peripheral regions that were close to the metal walls.

Supplementary Materials: The following supporting information can be downloaded at: https://www.mdpi.com/article/10.3390/ma18112548/s1, Figure S1: Effect of Mold Diameter on Depth of Cure.

Author Contributions: Conceptualization, R.B.P.; Data curation, A.G.; Investigation, A.G. and A.P.G.; Project administration, R.B.P.; Resources, R.B.P.; Software, R.B.P.; Supervision, R.B.P.; Visualization, A.P.G. and R.B.P.; Writing—original draft, A.G.; Writing—review and editing, A.G., A.P.G. and R.B.P. All authors have read and agreed to the published version of the manuscript.

Funding: The authors thank the Dalhousie Faculty of Dentistry Research Fund and Research Nova Scotia Intentional Initiative Award #2023-2885 for supporting this project.

Institutional Review Board Statement: Not applicable.

Informed Consent Statement: Not applicable.

Data Availability Statement: The data are available from the authors upon request.

Acknowledgments: The authors thank Ivoclar Vivadent AG for providing the Bluephase G4 and the resin-based composites used for this study. Also, the authors thank Cristiane Maucoski for her technical assistance with this project.

Conflicts of Interest: The authors declare that they have no conflicts of interest.

Abbreviations

The following abbreviations are used in this manuscript:

LCU	Light Curing Unit
RBC	Resin-based composite
DoC	Depth of Cure

References

1. FDI World Dental Federation. Dental amalgam phase down: Adopted by the FDI General Assembly: 7 September 2018, Buenos Aires, Argentina. *Int. Dent. J.* **2019**, *69*, 21–22. [CrossRef] [PubMed]
2. European Commission Welcomes Provisional Agreement to Ban All Remaining Intentional Uses of Toxic Mercury in the EU. Available online: https://ec.europa.eu/commission/presscorner/detail/en/IP_24_679 (accessed on 28 February 2024).
3. *ISO 4049*; Dentistry Polymer-Based Filling, Restorative Materials. International Standards Office: Geneva, Switzerland, 2019; p. 27.
4. Ferracane, J.L.; Hilton, T.J.; Stansbury, J.W.; Watts, D.C.; Silikas, N.; Ilie, N.; Heintze, S.; Cadenaro, M.; Hickel, R. Academy of Dental Materials guidance-Resin composites: Part II-Technique sensitivity (handling, polymerization, dimensional changes). *Dent. Mater.* **2017**, *33*, 1171–1191. [CrossRef] [PubMed]
5. Ilie, N.; Hilton, T.J.; Heintze, S.D.; Hickel, R.; Watts, D.C.; Silikas, N.; Stansbury, J.W.; Cadenaro, M.; Ferracane, J.L. Academy of Dental Materials guidance-Resin composites: Part I-Mechanical properties. *Dent. Mater.* **2017**, *33*, 880–894. [CrossRef]
6. Durner, J.; Obermaier, J.; Draenert, M.; Ilie, N. Correlation of the degree of conversion with the amount of elutable substances in nano-hybrid dental composites. *Dent. Mater.* **2012**, *28*, 1146–1153. [CrossRef]
7. Xu, X.; Sandras, D.A.; Burgess, J.O. Shear bond strength with increasing light-guide distance from dentin. *J. Esthet. Restor. Dent.* **2006**, *18*, 19–27; discussion 28. [CrossRef]
8. Hass, V.; Dobrovolski, M.; Zander-Grande, C.; Martins, G.C.; Gordillo, L.A.; Rodrigues Accorinte Mde, L.; Gomes, O.M.; Loguercio, A.D.; Reis, A. Correlation between degree of conversion, resin-dentin bond strength and nanoleakage of simplified etch-and-rinse adhesives. *Dent. Mater.* **2013**, *29*, 921–928. [CrossRef]
9. Vandewalle, K.S.; Ferracane, J.L.; Hilton, T.J.; Erickson, R.L.; Sakaguchi, R.L. Effect of energy density on properties and marginal integrity of posterior resin composite restorations. *Dent. Mater.* **2004**, *20*, 96–106. [CrossRef]
10. Ilie, N.; Schmalz, G.; Fujioka-Kobayashi, M.; Lussi, A.; Price, R.B. Correlation of the mechanical and biological response in light-cured RBCs to receiving a range of radiant exposures: Effect of violet light. *J. Dent.* **2021**, *105*, 103568. [CrossRef]

11. Ferracane, J.L.; Mitchem, J.C.; Condon, J.R.; Todd, R. Wear and marginal breakdown of composites with various degrees of cure. *J. Dent. Res.* **1997**, *76*, 1508–1516. [CrossRef]
12. Kleverlaan, C.J.; de Gee, A.J. Curing efficiency and heat generation of various resin composites cured with high-intensity halogen lights. *Eur. J. Oral Sci.* **2004**, *112*, 84–88. [CrossRef]
13. Fan, P.L.; Stanford, C.M.; Stanford, W.B.; Leung, R.; Stanford, J.W. Effects of backing reflectance and mold size on polymerization of photo-activated composite resin. *J. Dent. Res.* **1984**, *63*, 1245–1247. [CrossRef] [PubMed]
14. Harrington, E.; Wilson, H.J. Depth of cure of radiation-activated materials--effect of mould material and cavity size. *J. Dent.* **1993**, *21*, 305–311. [CrossRef] [PubMed]
15. Erickson, R.L.; Barkmeier, W.W. Curing characteristics of a composite. Part 2: The effect of curing configuration on depth and distribution of cure. *Dent. Mater.* **2014**, *30*, e134–e145. [CrossRef]
16. Erickson, R.L.; Barkmeier, W.W. Effect of mold diameter on the depth of cure of a resin-based composite material. *Eur. J. Oral Sci.* **2017**, *125*, 88–92. [CrossRef]
17. AlShaafi, M.M.; AlQussier, A.; AlQahtani, M.Q.; Price, R.B. Effect of Mold Type and Diameter on the Depth of Cure of Three Resin-Based Composites. *Oper. Dent.* **2018**, *43*, 520–529. [CrossRef]
18. Erickson, R.L.; Barkmeier, W.W. Comparisons of ISO depth of cure for a resin composite in stainless-steel and natural-tooth molds. *Eur. J. Oral Sci.* **2019**, *127*, 556–563. [CrossRef]
19. Vandewalle, K.S.; Roberts, H.W.; Rueggeberg, F.A. Power distribution across the face of different light guides and its effect on composite surface microhardness. *J. Esthet. Restor. Dent.* **2008**, *20*, 108–117; discussion 118. [CrossRef]
20. Shimokawa, C.; Turbino, M.L.; Giannini, M.; Braga, R.R.; Price, R.B. Effect of Curing Light and Exposure Time on the Polymerization of Bulk-Fill Resin-Based Composites in Molar Teeth. *Oper. Dent.* **2020**, *45*, E141–E155. [CrossRef]
21. Price, R.B.; Rueggeberg, F.A.; Harlow, J.; Sullivan, B. Effect of mold type, diameter, and uncured composite removal method on depth of cure. *Clin. Oral Investig.* **2016**, *20*, 1699–1707. [CrossRef]
22. Ribeiro, M.; Maucoski, C.; Price, R.B.; Soares, C.J. Effect of a 3-second Off-label Exposure on the Depth of Cure of Eight Resin-based Composites. *Oper. Dent.* **2024**, *49*, 421–431.
23. McCabe, J.F.; Carrick, T.E. Output from visible-light activation units and depth of cure of light-activated composites. *J. Dent. Res.* **1989**, *68*, 1534–1539. [CrossRef] [PubMed]
24. Asmussen, E.; Peutzfeldt, A. Polymer structure of a light-cured resin composite in relation to distance from the surface. *Eur. J. Oral Sci.* **2003**, *111*, 277–279. [CrossRef] [PubMed]
25. Cole, M.; Rueggeberg, F.A.; Looney, S.W.; Oxford, A.; Hassan, Z. Variation Comparison of Depth-of-Cure Between Scraping and Chemical Removal Methods. Abstract 2436. In Proceedings of the IADR General Session 2009, Miami, FL, USA, 1–4 April 2009.
26. Miletic, V.; Pongprueksa, P.; De Munck, J.; Brooks, N.R.; Van Meerbeek, B. Curing characteristics of flowable and sculptable bulk-fill composites. *Clin. Oral Investig.* **2017**, *21*, 1201–1212. [CrossRef]
27. Corciolani, G.; Vichi, A.; Davidson, C.L.; Ferrari, M. The influence of tip geometry and distance on light-curing efficacy. *Oper. Dent.* **2008**, *33*, 325–331. [CrossRef]
28. Comisi, J.C.; Price, R.B.; Kinley-Howard, K.; Maucoski, C.; Rader, E. Ability of Six Curing Lights to Photocure Four Resin-Based Composites in a MOD-Mold: A Double-Blind Study. *Eur. J. Prosthodont. Restor. Dent.* **2024**, *32*, 301–313.
29. Ash, M.M.; Nelson, S.J.; Ash, M.M. *Wheeler's Dental Anatomy, Physiology, and Occlusion*, 8th ed.; W.B. Saunders: Philadelphia, PA, USA, 2003; 523p.
30. Shimokawa, C.A.K.; Turbino, M.L.; Giannini, M.; Braga, R.R.; Price, R.B. Effect of light curing units on the polymerization of bulk fill resin-based composites. *Dent. Mater.* **2018**, *34*, 1211–1221. [CrossRef]
31. Hadis, M.A.; Shortall, A.C.; Palin, W.M. The power of light—From dental materials processing to diagnostics and therapeutics. *Biomater. Investig. Dent.* **2024**, *11*, 40308. [CrossRef]
32. Erickson, R.L.; Barkmeier, W.W.; Halvorson, R.H. Curing characteristics of a composite—Part 1: Cure depth relationship to conversion, hardness and radiant exposure. *Dent. Mater.* **2014**, *30*, e125–e133. [CrossRef]
33. Thomaidis, S.; Kampouropoulos, D.; Antoniadou, M.; Kakaboura, A. Evaluation of the Depth of Cure by Microhardness of Bulk-Fill Composites with Monowave and Polywave LED Light-Curing Units. *Appl. Sci.* **2024**, *14*, 11532. [CrossRef]
34. Contreras, S.C.M.; Jurema, A.L.B.; Claudino, E.S.; Bresciani, E.; Caneppele, T.M.F. Monowave and polywave light-curing of bulk-fill resin composites: Degree of conversion and marginal adaptation following thermomechanical aging. *Biomater. Investig. Dent.* **2021**, *8*, 72–78. [CrossRef]
35. Menees, T.S.; Lin, C.P.; Kojic, D.D.; Burgess, J.O.; Lawson, N.C. Depth of cure of bulk fill composites with monowave and polywave curing lights. *Am. J. Dent.* **2015**, *28*, 357–361.
36. *3s PowerCure: Scientific Documentation*; Ivoclar Vivadent AG Research and Development Scientific Services; Ivoclar Vivadent: Schaan, Liechtenstein, 2019.
37. *Aura Ultra Universal Bulk Fill Restorative Material Instructions for Use*; SDI Limited: Bayswater, VIC, Australia, 2016.

38. *Filtek One Bulk Fill Restorative: Technical Product Profile*; 3M Oral Care: St. Paul, MN, USA, 2016.
39. Hasslen, J.A.; Barkmeier, W.W.; Shaddy, R.S.; Little, J.R. Depth of cure of high-viscosity bulk-fill and conventional resin composites using varying irradiance exposures with a light-emitting diode curing unit. *J. Oral Sci.* **2019**, *61*, 425–430. [CrossRef]

materials

MDPI

Article

Chameleon Effect of Universal Shade Composite Polymers in Repairing CAD/CAM Lithium Disilicate

Gaetano Paolone *, Giacomo Collivasone, Niccolò De Masi, Alicia Heinichen, Katia Greco, Enrico Gherlone and Giuseppe Cantatore

Dental School, IRCCS San Raffaele Hospital, Vita-Salute University, 20132 Milan, Italy; g.collivasone@gmail.com (G.C.); niccolo_99@icloud.com (N.D.M.); a.heinichen@studenti.unisr.it (A.H.); katiagreco@libero.it (K.G.); gherlone.enrico@hsr.it (E.G.); cantatore.giuseppe@hsr.it (G.C.)
* Correspondence: paolone.gaetano@hsr.it

Abstract

The aim was to assess the blending effect of universal-shade resin-based composites (RBCs) (Omnichroma—OC; Clearfil Majesty Universal–CM; Venus Pearl—V; Transcend—T) used for repair for lithium disilicate blocks. Fifteen parallelepiped-shaped (10.5 × 10.5 × 3 mm) specimens with four cavities (3 mm in diameter and 2 mm in depth) were designed from lithium disilicate CAD/CAM blocks (CEREC Tessera HT A3) and milled. Specimens were then randomly divided into five groups based on the five resin composite materials for cavity restoration (n = 12): Group 1, control group (F); Group 2 (T); Group 3 (OC); Group 4 (V); and Group 5 (CM). After surface conditioning, composite resins were applied to the ceramic surface. Color measurements were taken with a colorimeter in the center of the resin restoration and on the CAD/CAM block. Tristimulus values were converted to CIELab color coordinates and color differences were expressed in ΔE_{00} units using the CIEDE-2000 formula. F showed significantly better color matching (ΔE_{00} = 2.51 ± 0.64) in comparison to single-shade RBCs except T (ΔE_{00} = 2.55 ± 0.64). All groups exceeded perceptibility and acceptability thresholds. The control group presented higher color matching than the single shade universal composites except for Transcend.

Keywords: chameleon effect; universal shades; CAD/CAM; lithium disilicate; composite; repair; color adjustment potential

1. Introduction

The introduction of the acid-etch technique in 1955 by Michael Buonocore [1], the bisphenol A-glycidyl methacrylate (Bis-GMA) by Dr. Bowen [2] in the early 1960s, and subsequently, the launching of the first commercial resin-based composite (RBC) set a milestone for adhesive dentistry. Ever since, constant modifications have been made to improve the properties of RBCs. Nowadays, clinicians have a plethora of composites with enhanced physical properties used to functionally and esthetically restore both anterior and posterior teeth. The tooth is composed of different tissues and the shade derives from the combination between them and light. Dentin is the dental tissue mainly responsible for its color [3], while enamel is a colorless and translucent tissue that acts as a filter [4], since the orientation of enamel rods causes light to be scattered. When a resin restoration is placed, a complex color interaction between dental tissues and RBCs takes place. According to several factors, RBCs may have a variable degree of camouflage with the dental substrate. Hall and Kafalias [5] reported this phenomenon as the "chameleon effect". In the literature, other terms such as "color assimilation" [6], "blending effect" (BE) [7], or "color adjustment potential" (CAP) [8] are also used to describe the ability to blend with the surrounding tooth substrate. In the last decades, dental companies have launched different composite shades with similar optical properties to enamel and dentin, introducing composite layering techniques [9–12]. Clinicians need to stratify different restorative material to an adequate thickness and position to create an almost imperceptible restoration [13]. Koi et al. [14] reported that mastering the different layering concepts is time-consuming and a compelling task that depends on clinical expertise. Recently, to simplify clinical protocols, the industry has aimed to reduce the number of shades and universal shades have been introduced [14,15]. As reported by Altınışık and Özyurt [16], these new composites have the advantage of being able to simulate all shades of tooth color using only a single shade. Hence, manufacturers claim that these universal composite resins are able to have a true chameleon effect [17,18]. Perdigão et al. [19] reported that these new materials not only offer tremendous advantages but also revolutionize their promising use in clinical practice, particularly when compared to materials that require multiple shades to accomplish a successful restoration. Ceramics can also address the demands for cosmetic dentistry, as they are considered the material closest to dental structures. Thanks to their excellent mechanical, chemical, and optical properties [20,21], they can mimic the natural appearance of teeth. Above all, they offer high biocompatibility and stability [22]. To date, silicates, and in particular lithium disilicate, are one of the most widespread and versatile dental ceramics used [23]. However, two major drawbacks have to be considered, which are production costs and cyclic fatigue [24]. Common complications comprise chipping, cracking, and fracture [25–27], and represent an esthetical and functional problem for patients [28]. RBCs are the most widely used material for repair as they avoid the expense and time of remaking of ceramic [29]. The use of simplified restorative procedures, including universal composites, could facilitate clinicians' procedures and increase the longevity of ceramic frameworks. The aim of this study was, therefore, to assess the chameleon effect of four universal shades used for repair of lithium disilicate prosthetic elements. The null hypothesis was that there is no difference in the ability to blend in for universal composites, compared to conventional RBCs.

2. Materials and Methods

Lithium disilicate CAD/CAM blocks (CEREC Tessera® HT A3 C14, shade A3, Dentsply Sirona, Charlotte, CN, USA) were milled to create four cavities with a depth of 2 mm and a diameter of 3 mm. The specimens were then filled with the tested materials ($n = 12$). The characteristics and composition of the tested materials used in this study are presented in Table 1.

2.1. Specimen Preparation

An original experimental set was created to perform this study. A total of 15 parallelepiped-shaped specimens (10.5 × 10.5 × 3 mm) with four cavities (∅ 3 mm × depth 2 mm) were designed with an online software (Tinkercad®, Autodesk, San Francisco, CA, USA), and the obtained standard tessellation language (STL) file was imported into the InLab® CAM (Dentsply Sirona, Charlotte, NC, USA) software program (Figure 1). Each specimen was milled (Figure 2) with Cylinder Pointed Burs 12S and Step Burs 12S (Dentsply Sirona, Charlotte, NC, USA) in a precision chairside wet milling machine, CEREC® MC XL (Dentsply Sirona, Charlotte, NC, USA). For each specimen, a new set of burs was used, the water tank was pulled out from the milling unit, the filter was replaced, and new distilled water and lubricant (DENTATEC CEREC/inLab; Dentsply Sirona, Charlotte, NC, USA) were filled into the tank. The specimens were consequently subjected to the crystallization process, as indicated by the manufacturer, in a SpeedFire® furnace (Dentsply Sirona, Charlotte, NC, USA).

Table 1. Manufacturers' information about the RBCs.

Materials	Manufacturer	Shade	Monomers	Filler Size/Content	Filler [*w*/*v*%]
Omnichroma® (OC) G3	Tokuyama Dental Corporation, Tokyo, Japan	Universal	UDMA, TEGDMA	SiO_2, ZrO_2, CF	79/68
Transcend® (T) G2	Ultradent Products Inc., South Jordan, UT, USA	UB	5 different resin monomers described as functional methacrylates	Five different types of silicate fillers, ranging in size from 5 nm to 3 μm	77.5/na
Venus Pearl® (V) G4	Heraeaus Kulzer, Hanau, Germany	One	UDMA, TCD-DI-HEA, TEGDMA	Ba-Al-B-F-Si, PPF, SiO_2	75/59
Clearfil Majesty Universal® (CM) G5	Kuraray Noritake Dental, Osaka, Japan	Universal	Bis-GMA, Hydrophobic aliphatic dimethacrylate, Hydrophobic aromatic dimethacrylate, di-camphorquinone	Silinated barium glass filler	78/66
Forma® (F) G1	Ultradent Products Inc, SP, Brazil	A3B	Bis-GMA, Bis-EMA, TEGDMA, BHT, PEGDMA, UDMA, ytterbium trifluoride	Silane-treated ceramic, silane-treated silica, silane-treated silica–zirconium oxide and barium glass	67/na
CEREC Tessera® HT	Dentsply Sirona, Charlotte, NC, USA	A3	90% lithium disilicate ($Li_2Si_2O_5$), 5% virgilite ($Li_{0.5}Al_{0.5}Si_{2.5}O_6$) 5% Li_3PO_4		

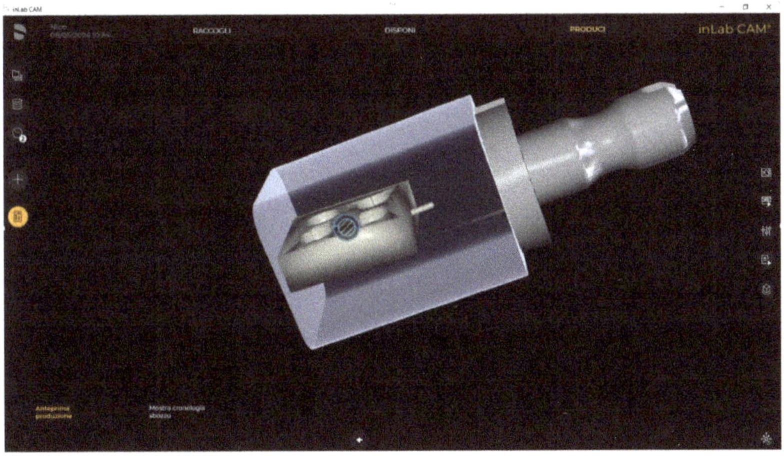

Figure 1. Preview of the specimens' design.

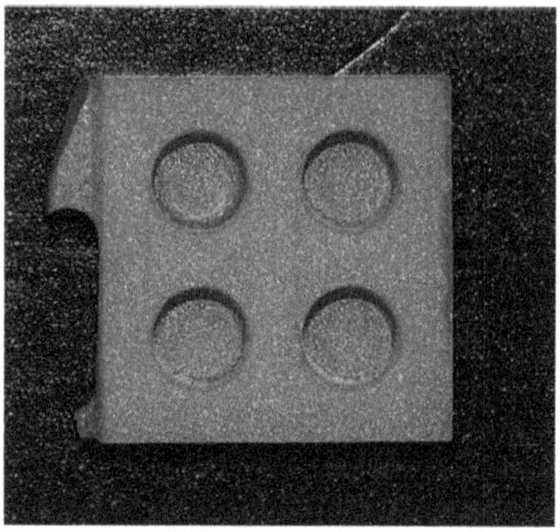

Figure 2. Preparation of the specimen.

2.2. Surface Treatment

The inner surfaces of each cavity were etched using 5% hydrofluoric acid (HF; IPS Ceramic Etching Gel, Ivoclar, Schaan, Liechtenstein) for 20 s, rinsed with water for 30 s, and then dried with air blowing. Then, silane coupling agent (Silane, Ultradent, South Jordan, UT, USA) was applied for 1 min, followed by air blowing. The universal adhesive system Futurabond U (Voco, GmbH, Cuxhaven, Germany) was applied to the cavities with the aid of a microbrush, using friction movement on the ceramic structure for 20 s. A brief jet of air was then applied over the bonding agent for 5 s before the adhesive system was light cured for 20 s using an LED curing unit (LCU; VALO Corded, Ultradent, UT, USA) with an irradiance of 1200 mW/cm^2. The cavities were filled with the investigated RBCs (n = 12), applying two increments. The last increment was covered with a Mylar strip and pressed using a glass slide with a constant 1 kg pressure to obtain a flat surface. The composite restorations were polymerized for 20 s with the LED held centered over each cavity. After curing, restorations were polished by the same operator using Sof-Lex DiscsTM (3M ESPE, St. Paul, MI, USA). A medium, fine, and extra-fine grit sequence of Sof-Lex was used sequentially with mild hand pressure. A new set of discs was used for every specimen.

2.3. Instrumental Evaluation

Color parameters were measured, after 72 h of storage in distilled water, using a professional benchtop colorimeter, Easy Color (SmartVision, Udine, Italy) (Figure 3).

The settings were as follows: illuminant: *D*; and temperature: 50 with a neutral grey background (ISO/TR 28642 [30]). White and black calibration was performed as suggested by the manufacturer at the beginning of the test and after each group was completed.

Measurements were performed at two points:

- At the center of resin composite restoration;
- At the center of the CAD/CAM block at an equidistant position to the 4 cavities.

Measurements were repeated by the same operator three times for each composite restoration and specimen, and the average value over the three measurements was calculated. The CIE XYZ tristimulus values were converted to CIE L*a*b* parameters using a dedicated software (SmartVision Easy Color, Udine, Italy): L* refers to luminosity (L* = 0 = black; L* = 100 = white), a* indicates the chroma on the red–green axis (a* $\geq$ 0 = red and a* $\leq$ 0 = green), and b* the chroma on the yellow–blue axis

($b^* \geq 0$ = yellow; $b^* \leq 0$ =blue). Color differences were expressed in ΔE_{00} units using the CIEDE 2000 color difference according to the following equation [31–33]:

$$\Delta E_{00} = [\left(\frac{\Delta L'}{k_L S_L}\right)^2 + \left(\frac{\Delta C'}{k_C S_C}\right)^2 + \left(\frac{\Delta H'}{k_H S_H}\right)^2 + R_T\left(\frac{\Delta C'}{k_C S_C}\right)\left(\frac{\Delta H'}{k_H S_H}\right)]^{\frac{1}{2}} \quad (1)$$

where $\Delta L'$, $\Delta C'$, and $\Delta H'$ are the differences in lightness, chroma, and hue, respectively, for a pair of points. The weighting functions (SL, SC, and SH) adjust the total color difference for variation in the location of the color difference pair in the L', a', and b' coordinates. The parametric factors (k_L, k_C, and k_H) were set to 1. The three ΔE_{00} values obtained for each tested material were averaged to obtain one mean ΔE_{00} value for each RBC. Color adaptability was assessed based on the color differences between the lithium disilicate block and composites across the threshold of 50%:50% perceptibility (PT) and 50:50% acceptability (AT) according to ISO/TR 28642:2016. The values $\Delta E_{00} = 0.8$ and $\Delta E_{00} = 1.8$ were reported as the 50:50% perceptibility threshold (PT) and 50:50% acceptability threshold (AT) [34].

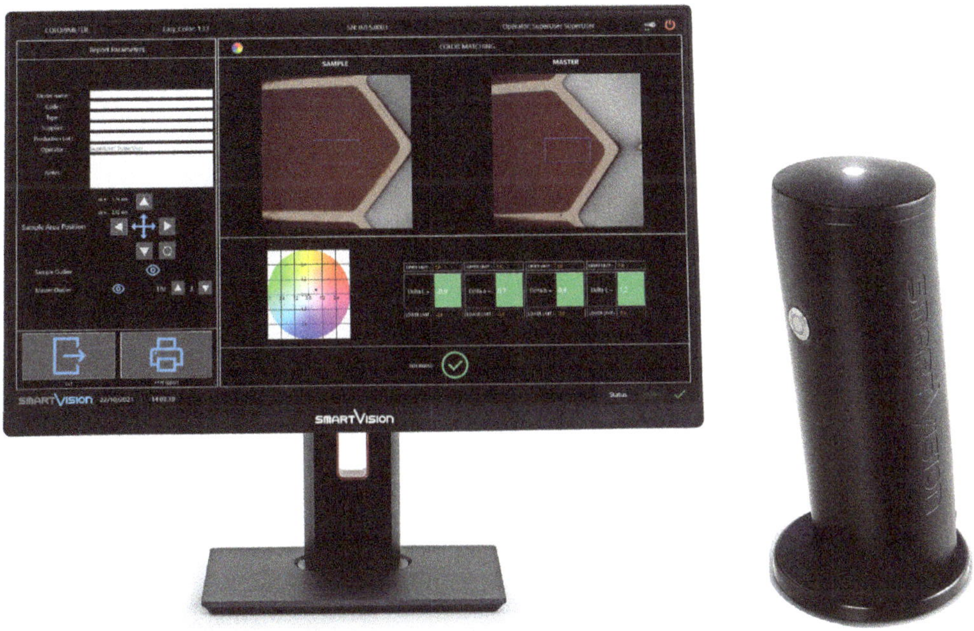

Figure 3. The professional benchtop colorimeter used in this study.

2.4. Statistical Analysis

The normal distribution of data was verified using the Shapiro–Wilk test, and the homogeneity of variance was assessed using the Brown–Forsythe test. Mean values were compared to determine which of the five tested materials was the closest match using a one-way analysis of variance (ANOVA) test. All analyses were performed with the statistical platform STATA (STATA, v12.0, StataCorp, College Station, TX, USA). For the current study, the level of significance (α) is 5%. Hence, $p \leq 0.05$ was considered significant.

3. Results

One-way analysis of variance (ANOVA) showed significant differences ($p < 0.05$) in the ability of materials to blend with the substrate. Table 2 and Figure 4 both present the mean color differences (ΔE_{00}) and standard deviations (SDs) between the baseline lithium disilicate block and restored cavities for each group. All restorations with the tested materials presented color difference levels above the acceptable threshold (AT = 1.8). Among the study groups, CM showed the highest ΔE_{00} (5.53 ± 0.60), while F, a multi-shade RBC, showed the lowest (2.51 ± 0.79). For all other groups, ΔE_{00} ranged from 2.55 ± 0.64 to 5.34 ± 0.76, with significant differences ($p < 0.05$). The results showed there was a statistically significant difference between the control group G1 and the tested groups G3, G4, and G5 ($p < 0.05$). Pairwise comparisons showed significant differences ($p < 0.05$) between G3 and G4, between G3 and G5, between G2 and G4, between G2 and G5, and between G4 and G5. No significant difference was found between the control group G1 and G2 and between G2 and G3 ($p > 0.05$).

Table 2. Mean of colors difference values (ΔE_{00}) and SDs for the five composite materials tested in the study. The same letters (A to D) represent no statistically significant differences ($p > 0.05$).

Groups	ΔE_{00} Mean and Standard Deviation
G1 (F; control)	2.51 ± 0.79 ^{A}
G2 (T)	2.55 ± 0.64 ^{AB}
G3 (OC)	3.41 ± 0.92 ^{B}
G4 (V)	5.34 ± 0.76 ^{C}
G5 (CM)	5.53 ± 0.60 ^{Ds}

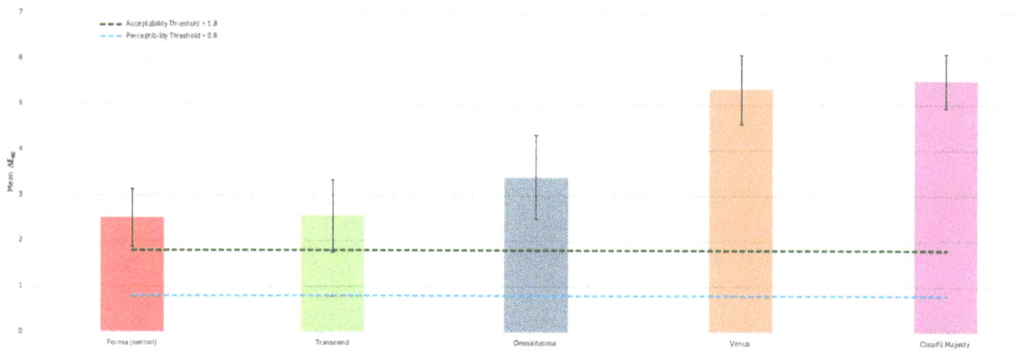

Figure 4. Column chart showing the mean ΔE_{00} for the tested materials. The black vertical lines represent the standard deviation for each group. The green dashed line represents the acceptability threshold ($\Delta E_{00} = 1.8$) and the blue dashed line represents the perceptibility threshold ($\Delta E_{00} = 0.8$). Shorter columns show better integration.

A clear trend emerged: materials with defined shades or with fillers chemically similar to the lithium disilicate substrate (e.g., Transcend) tended to show better color matching. All groups, however, exceeded the clinical acceptability threshold, underscoring limitations in the universal shade concept under these testing conditions. No anomalies or outliers were observed, and data showed normal distribution and homoscedasticity.

4. Discussion

To reduce operative time and simplify clinical procedures, which are often too technique-sensitive, the industry has invested in developing single-shade universal composites [8]. Manufacturers claim that these new composites can mimic the color of the surrounding tooth regardless of its shade. The objective of this study was to instrumentally evaluate the chameleon effect of four commercially available universal shade composites compared to a multi-shade resin-based composite (RBC) used for the repair of lithium disilicate prosthetic elements. The null hypothesis was rejected, as statistically significant differences were observed between the control and the tested groups. The results showed that the ΔE_{00} values for all groups exceeded the perceptibility (PT) and acceptability (AT) thresholds, indicating that the shade mismatches were not only perceptible but also clinically unacceptable. Among all tested materials, Forma (F) demonstrated significantly better color adjustment (ΔE_{00} = 2.51) than the universal composites, except for Transcend (T) (ΔE_{00} = 2.55). The average ΔE_{00} value of the control group was closer to the acceptability threshold than those of the universal shade composites. De Abreu et al. [35] and Korkut et al. [36] experimented on the color adjustment potential of composites in class III cavities and class I cavities, respectively. In both these in-vitro studies, RBCs with a defined shade (e.g., A1, A2, A3, etc.) showed better color matching. The results reported in our study are consistent with their findings. Forma's superior blending may be attributed to two main factors: shade selection and translucency. Paravina et al. [7] determined that the BE increases when there is less color difference between the RBCs and the surrounding structure. Amid the materials tested, the control group was the only one with a defined shade (A3) that matched the substrate. The use of specific color pigments may have enhanced the blending capability of the control group. Villarroel et al. [37] have shown that translucency plays a key role in the perceived color of a restoration. Various factors [38] can influence translucency and consequently, the blending behavior of resin composites. These include material thickness, shade, background environment, resin matrix composition, filler content and size [39], and refractive index (RI) [40]. The RI of a material affects light propagation and thus the perceived color of the restoration. A close match in RI between the resin and surrounding tooth structure results in minimal light scattering [40,41], leading to higher translucency and improved blending. Conversely, a mismatch in RI can cause shadow-like effects at the restoration margins due to destructive light interference between materials with different RI values [37,42]. Therefore, to achieve a natural appearance, dental composites should have an RI as close as possible to that of natural enamel [37,43], which has a reported mean RI of 1.631 [44]. The average RI of lithium disilicate is 1.55 in the visible light spectrum [45], while that of Bis-GMA is 1.54 [46]. This close match between the refractive indices of lithium disilicate and Forma may partly explain the superior color matching observed with Forma. However, CM also contains Bis-GMA, yet it exhibited the lowest chameleon effect. The RI of a resin composite is influenced by both the type of resin matrix and the inorganic fillers added [46]. Since F is the only material in this study that includes the specialized filler ytterbium trifluoride—whose RI is very close to that of resin monomers (1.49–1.56) [47]—it is likely that the presence of this filler contributes significantly to its enhanced translucency. Paravina et al. [7] reported that the BE increases with greater translucency, supporting the hypothesis that the addition of ytterbium trifluoride may explain Forma's superior chameleon effect in this study. Nevertheless, RI is not the only factor to consider in achieving esthetic restorations. Proper thickness is equally important. A linear decrease in RI with increasing specimen thickness was observed by Son et al. [48]. Further research varying the thickness of single-shade specimens could help quantify the impact of this variable on RI. Among the universal shades, Transcend (T) showed the lowest ΔE_{00} value, while CM showed the highest. The high color match of T may be attributed to its inclusion of five different types of silicate fillers—chemically similar to those in lithium disilicate—potentially allowing a more mimetic repair. Conversely, CM's poorer color match could be due to its larger filler particles (mean size of 1.5 μm), which tend to scatter more light and reduce transmittance [49,50]. OC, in comparison, showed a lower blending effect than T, though without statistically significant differences. OC does not contain Bis-GMA in its resin matrix and incorporates uniformly sized 260 nm spherical silicon/zirconium dioxide fillers. It also features a structural color-based shading system, meaning it achieves color through the physical structure of its fillers rather than through added pigments. This may have affected its color blending performance compared to the other materials evaluated.

Our findings contrast with those of Pereira Sanchez et al. [8], who reported a greater color-matching ability for OC. However, their study evaluated OC in posterior occlusal restorations and used the CIELab formula, which may account for the discrepancy. Recent studies have concluded that the CIEDE2000 formula more accurately reflects human visual perception than the traditional CIELab color difference metric [51–54]. This difference may account for the discrepancies between studies. Conversely, our findings align with those of Iyer et al. [55]. They found that OC exhibited inferior color-matching ability compared to a resin composite with a defined shade. They also observed that OC visually matched better with lighter shades. Islam et al. reported [56] that OC blended more effectively with shades such as B1, A2, and B2 of CharmFil Plus (CP) and Filtek Universal Restorative (3M), but showed greater contrast with darker shades like A3 and A3.5. Since shade A3 was used in our study, this could partially explain OC's lower CAP. Akgul et al. [57] demonstrated that increasing the cavity size enhanced OC's blending effect, likely due to changes in the optical behavior of surrounding tooth structures. They concluded that 3.0 mm restorations achieved better color matching than 2.0 mm ones. In our experiment, standardized cavities with a depth of 2 mm and diameter of 3 mm were selected to ensure complete curing of the RBCs. Further studies varying cavity depth could help determine whether restoration size influences the blending performance of universal shade composites. Additionally, the study by Korkut et al. [36] reported improved CAP of OC and Essentia Universal after two weeks compared to the baseline measurements. These findings underscore the need for long-term evaluations to assess the durability of the chameleon effect. Surface treatment may also affect the optical blending behavior of universal shades. In the study by Karabulut et al. [58], a higher color difference for OC in Sylc-treated Empress blocks was observed, while Essentia Universal exhibited greater color shifts in Sylc-treated Cerasmart270 CAD blocks. The authors attributed these differences to the adhesion of Sylc particles, which may interact differently with various chromatic technologies. Therefore, further investigation into how surface treatments influence color performance is warranted. Similarly, the type of adhesive system can impact the final shade of the restoration. According to Schneider et al. [59], adhesives may alter color parameters, particularly along the a and b axes, largely due to their chemical composition. Oxidative reactions involving Camphorquinone and amine components—such as those found in Futurabond U—can lead to darkening and increased yellowing over time. Beyond differences in filler content and translucency, deeper material science factors may explain the superior blending of certain RBCs. One critical aspect is the homogeneity of the resin–filler interface: a well-integrated interface minimizes internal light scattering and promotes more uniform light transmission. In composites with nano- or submicron fillers, such as Transcend, light scattering may occur in the Rayleigh regime, where intensity is inversely proportional to the fourth power of the wavelength [60]. This selective wavelength scattering can enhance visual blending with adjacent structures.

Moreover, the stability and distribution of filler particles within the resin matrix influence not only the mechanical properties but also the optical phase continuity—governing how light transitions between resin and filler phases [60,61]. Composites with high optical phase continuity, minimal refractive index mismatches, and optimized filler–resin coupling are more likely to deliver superior optical blending [62]. These findings suggest that the chameleon effect is influenced by both translucency and the nanoscale architecture of the composite.

When performing repairs of lithium disilicate restorations, clinicians should be aware that not all universal shade composites provide comparable blending performance. Materials with defined shades—such as Forma (A3)—demonstrated superior optical integration due to better shade matching and refractive index compatibility. Among universal composites, those containing finer filler particles and chemically similar filler compositions to lithium disilicate, such as Transcend, may provide better esthetic results. Clinicians are advised to consider multiple factors when selecting a repair composite, including the shade of the ceramic substrate, the translucency of the composite, and the material's refractive properties [63]. Whenever possible, visual evaluation and shade matching before initiating the repair procedure are recommended to optimize esthetic outcomes.

The clinical implications of the current study are as follows: using defined-shade composites in shade-specific repairs improves the esthetic integration of the restoration; although universal composites offer workflow simplicity, they may not meet patients' esthetic expectations in visible areas; and visual shade selection and pre-curing evaluation are recommended to confirm the suitability of the selected composite.

This study evaluated the chameleon effect of universal shade composites in repairing CAD/CAM lithium disilicate restorations; however, several limitations should be acknowledged. The in vitro nature of the research does not fully replicate clinical conditions, where factors such as saliva, observer variability, absence of aging and thermal cycling, temperature variations, and occlusal forces may affect the blending ability and long-term stability of the restorations. Moreover, only one shade of lithium disilicate (HT A3) was tested, whereas the color adaptation of universal composites could vary depending on the background shade and translucency. Another limitation is the short-term assessment, as color measurements were performed immediately after restoration placement, without considering aging effects such as wear, staining, and potential discoloration over time. To address the limitations inherent in this in vitro, short-term study, future research should incorporate clinically relevant aging simulations and visual assessments. Specifically, thermocycling and artificial staining protocols could be applied to evaluate the durability of the chameleon effect under intraoral-like conditions. Additionally, long-term monitoring of color stability over periods of 1–6 months would help quantify time-dependent changes in blending behavior. Including subjective visual assessments by trained evaluators—alongside instrumental colorimetry—would offer a more comprehensive evaluation of esthetic performance. These strategies would help bridge the gap between laboratory findings and real-world clinical applicability. Further studies are warranted to explore the impact of cavity depth and size on the blending effect, as well as investigate different surface treatment protocols and adhesive systems that may influence optical behavior. Additionally, color assessment in this study was instrumentally performed, without accounting for human visual perception, which plays a key role in clinical esthetics. Incorporating both objective and subjective evaluations would provide a more comprehensive understanding of color matching.

Long-term clinical trials are essential to validate the findings from in vitro experiments and assess the durability and overall performance of universal shade composites in real-world conditions.

5. Conclusions

Within the limitations of the present study, it can be concluded that among universal composites, Transcend approached the performance of the multi-shade material but still exceeded the acceptability threshold under these test conditions. These outcomes indicate that universal shade composites do not uniformly achieve reliable blending with ceramic substrates. Clinicians should consider material composition and optical compatibility when esthetics are critical.

Author Contributions: Conceptualization, G.P.; Methodology, N.D.M.; Software, N.D.M.; Validation, N.D.M., E.G. and G.C. (Giuseppe Cantatore); Formal analysis, G.P.; Resources, K.G.; Data curation, G.C. (Giacomo Collivasone) and G.C. (Giuseppe Cantatore); Writing—original draft, A.H.; Writing—review & editing, G.P.; Visualization, E.G. and K.G.; Supervision, G.P.; Project administration, G.P. All authors have read and agreed to the published version of the manuscript.

Funding: This research received no external funding.

Institutional Review Board Statement: Not applicable.

Informed Consent Statement: Not applicable.

Data Availability Statement: The raw data supporting the conclusions of this article will be made available by the authors on request.

Conflicts of Interest: The authors declare no conflicts of interest.

Abbreviations

The following abbreviations are used in this manuscript:

RBCs	Resin-based composites
OC	Omnichroma
CM	Clearfil Majesty Universal
V	Venus Pearl
T	Transcend
F	Forma
BE	Blending effect
CAP	Color adjustment potential
HF	Hydrofluoric acid
LCU	LED curing unit
AT	Acceptability threshold
PT	Perceptibility threshold
SDs	Standard deviations
RI	Refractive index

References

1. Buonocore, M.G. A Simple Method of Increasing the Adhesion of Acrylic Filling Materials to Enamel Surfaces. *J. Dent. Res.* **1955**, *34*, 849–853. [CrossRef] [PubMed]
2. Bowen, R.L. Properties of a Silica-Reinforced Polymer for Dental Restorations. *J. Am. Dent. Assoc.* **1963**, *66*, 57–64. [CrossRef] [PubMed]
3. ten Bosch, J.J.; Coops, J.C. Tooth Color and Reflectance as Related to Light Scattering and Enamel Hardness. *J. Dent. Res.* **1995**, *74*, 374–380. [CrossRef] [PubMed]
4. Orban, J.B.; Sicher, H.; Bhaskar, S.N. *Orban's Oral Histology and Embryology*, 7th ed.; The C.V. Mosby Company: St. Louis, MO, USA, 1972; ISBN 978-0-8016-4607-2.
5. Hall, N.R.; Kafalias, M.C. Composite Colour Matching: The Development and Evaluation of a Restorative Colour Matching System. *Aust. Prosthodont. J.* **1991**, *5*, 47–52.

6. Lee, Y.-K.; Yu, B.; Zhao, G.-F.; Lim, J.I. Color Assimilation of Resin Composites with Adjacent Color According to the Distance. *J. Esthet. Restor. Dent.* **2015**, *27* (Suppl. 1), S24–S32. [CrossRef]
7. Paravina, R.D.; Westland, S.; Imai, F.H.; Kimura, M.; Powers, J.M. Evaluation of Blending Effect of Composites Related to Restoration Size. *Dent. Mater.* **2006**, *22*, 299–307. [CrossRef]
8. Pereira Sanchez, N.; Powers, J.M.; Paravina, R.D. Instrumental and Visual Evaluation of the Color Adjustment Potential of Resin Composites. *J. Esthet. Restor. Dent.* **2019**, *31*, 465–470. [CrossRef]
9. Fahl, N.; Denehy, G.E.; Jackson, R.D. Protocol for Predictable Restoration of Anterior Teeth with Composite Resins. *Pract. Periodontics Aesthet. Dent.* **1995**, *7*, 13–21, quiz 22.
10. Dietschi, D.; Dietschi, J.M. Current Developments in Composite Materials and Techniques. *Pract. Periodontics Aesthet. Dent.* **1996**, *8*, 603–613, quiz 614.
11. Dietschi, D. Layering Concepts in Anterior Composite Restorations. *J. Adhes. Dent.* **2001**, *3*, 71–80.
12. Magne, P.; Holz, J. Stratification of Composite Restorations: Systematic and Durable Replication of Natural Aesthetics. *Pract. Periodontics Aesthet. Dent.* **1996**, *8*, 61–68, quiz 70. [PubMed]
13. Paolone, G. Direct Composites in Anteriors: A Matter of Substrate. *Int. J. Esthet. Dent.* **2017**, *12*, 468–481. [PubMed]
14. Koi, K.; Amaya-Pajares, S.P.; Kawashima, S.; Arora, G.; Ferracane, J.; Watanabe, H. The Color-Matching Ability of Single-Shade Universal Composites in Extracted Human Teeth. *J. Esthet. Restor. Dent.* **2025**, *37*, 456–464. [CrossRef]
15. Bisharah, W.F.; Zahran, A.S.; Rajeh, M.T.; AbdelAleem, N.A. In Vitro Comparison of Color Matching: Universal Shade Composite Resin vs Multi-Shade Conventional Composite. *J. Contemp. Dent. Pract.* **2024**, *25*, 1039–1044. [CrossRef]
16. Altınışık, H.; Özyurt, E. Instrumental and Visual Evaluation of the Color Adjustment Potential of Different Single-Shade Resin Composites to Human Teeth of Various Shades. *Clin. Oral. Investig.* **2023**, *27*, 889–896. [CrossRef]
17. Ismail, E.H.; Paravina, R.D. Color Adjustment Potential of Resin Composites: Optical Illusion or Physical Reality, a Comprehensive Overview. *J. Esthet. Restor. Dent.* **2022**, *34*, 42–54. [CrossRef]
18. Floriani, F.; Tsujimoto, A.; Jurado, C.A.; Oliveira, D.; Rojas-Rueda, S.; Lopes, G.C. Color Match and Stability of Single-Shade Resin-Based Composites before and after Artificial Aging. *Am. J. Dent.* **2024**, *37*, 297–302.
19. Perdigão, J.; Araujo, E.; Ramos, R.Q.; Gomes, G.; Pizzolotto, L. Adhesive Dentistry: Current Concepts and Clinical Considerations. *J. Esthet. Restor. Dent.* **2021**, *33*, 51–68. [CrossRef]
20. Magne, P.; Versluis, A.; Douglas, W.H. Rationalization of Incisor Shape: Experimental-Numerical Analysis. *J. Prosthet. Dent.* **1999**, *81*, 345–355. [CrossRef]
21. Bajraktarova-Valjakova, E.; Korunoska-Stevkovska, V.; Kapusevska, B.; Gigovski, N.; Bajraktarova-Misevska, C.; Grozdanov, A. Contemporary Dental Ceramic Materials, A Review: Chemical Composition, Physical and Mechanical Properties, Indications for Use. *Open Access Maced. J. Med. Sci.* **2018**, *6*, 1742–1755. [CrossRef]
22. van Noort, R. *Introduction to Dental Materials*, 3rd ed.; Mosby Elsevier: St Louis, MO, USA, 2007; ISBN 978-0-7234-3404-7.
23. Zarone, F.; Di Mauro, M.I.; Ausiello, P.; Ruggiero, G.; Sorrentino, R. Current Status on Lithium Disilicate and Zirconia: A Narrative Review. *BMC Oral Health* **2019**, *19*, 134. [CrossRef] [PubMed]
24. Zhang, Y.; Sailer, I.; Lawn, B.R. Fatigue of Dental Ceramics. *J. Dent.* **2013**, *41*, 1135–1147. [CrossRef] [PubMed]
25. Alsarani, M.; Souza, G.D.; Rizkalla, A.; El-Mowafy, O. Influence of Crown Design and Material on Chipping-Resistance of All-Ceramic Molar Crowns: An in Vitro Study. *Dent. Med. Probl.* **2018**, *55*, 35–42. [CrossRef]
26. Dhima, M.; Carr, A.B.; Salinas, T.J.; Lohse, C.; Berglund, L.; Nan, K.-A. Evaluation of Fracture Resistance in Aqueous Environment under Dynamic Loading of Lithium Disilicate Restorative Systems for Posterior Applications. Part 2. *J. Prosthodont.* **2014**, *23*, 353–357. [CrossRef]
27. Hickel, R.; Brüshaver, K.; Ilie, N. Repair of Restorations--Criteria for Decision Making and Clinical Recommendations. *Dent. Mater.* **2013**, *29*, 28–50. [CrossRef]
28. Garbelotto, L.G.D.; Fukushima, K.A.; Özcan, M.; Cesar, P.F.; Volpato, C.A.M. Chipping of Veneering Ceramic on a Lithium Disilicate Anterior Single Crown: Description of Repair Method and a Fractographic Failure Analysis. *J. Esthet. Restor. Dent.* **2019**, *31*, 299–303. [CrossRef]
29. Reston, E.G.; Filho, S.C.; Arossi, G.; Cogo, R.B.; dos Santos Rocha, C.; Closs, L.Q. Repairing Ceramic Restorations: Final Solution or Alternative Procedure? *Oper. Dent.* **2008**, *33*, 461–466. [CrossRef]
30. *ISO 28642: 2011*; Dentistry—Guidance on Color Measurement. International Organization for Standardization: Geneva, Switzerland, 2025.
31. *CIE Publication 15-2*; Colorimetry; CIE Central Bureau: Vienna, Austria, 1986.
32. *ISO 11664-4: 2008(E)/CIE S 014-4/E:2007CIE*; Colorimetry—Part 4: CIE 1976 L*a*b* Colour Space. International Organization for Standardization: Geneva, Switzerland, 2008; p. 1976.
33. *ISO/CIE 11664-6:2014*; Colorimetry—Part 6: CIEDE2000 Color-Difference Formula. CIE Central Bureau: Vienna, Austria, 2014.

34. Paravina, R.D.; Ghinea, R.; Herrera, L.J.; Bona, A.D.; Igiel, C.; Linninger, M.; Sakai, M.; Takahashi, H.; Tashkandi, E.; Mal Perez, M.D. Color Difference Thresholds in Dentistry. *J. Esthet. Restor. Dent.* **2015**, *27* (Suppl. 1), S1–S9. [CrossRef]
35. de Abreu, J.L.B.; Sampaio, C.S.; Benalcázar Jalkh, E.B.; Hirata, R. Analysis of the Color Matching of Universal Resin Composites in Anterior Restorations. *J. Esthet. Restor. Dent.* **2021**, *33*, 269–276. [CrossRef]
36. Korkut, B.; Çiğdem, H.; Ezgi Tüter, B.; Funda, Y. The Assessment of Color Adjustment Potentials for Monoshade Universal Composites. *De Gruyter* **2023**, *30*, 590–604. [CrossRef]
37. Villarroel, M.; Fahl, N.; De Sousa, A.M.; De Oliveira, O.B. Direct Esthetic Restorations Based on Translucency and Opacity of Composite Resins. *J. Esthet. Restor. Dent.* **2011**, *23*, 73–87. [CrossRef] [PubMed]
38. Powers, J.M.; Dennison, J.B.; Lepeak, P.J. Parameters That Affect the Color of Direct Restorative Resins. *J. Dent. Res.* **1978**, *57*, 876–880. [CrossRef] [PubMed]
39. Lim, Y.-K.; Lee, Y.-K.; Lim, B.-S.; Rhee, S.-H.; Yang, H.-C. Influence of Filler Distribution on the Color Parameters of Experimental Resin Composites. *Dent. Mater.* **2008**, *24*, 67–73. [CrossRef] [PubMed]
40. Ota, M.; Ando, S.; Endo, H.; Ogura, Y.; Miyazaki, M.; Hosoya, Y. Influence of Refractive Index on Optical Parameters of Experimental Resin Composites. *Acta Odontol. Scand.* **2012**, *70*, 362–367. [CrossRef]
41. Lee, Y.-K. Influence of Scattering/Absorption Characteristics on the Color of Resin Composites. *Dent. Mater.* **2007**, *23*, 124–131. [CrossRef]
42. Beolchi, R.S.; Mehta, D.; Pelissier, B.; Gênova, L.A.; Freitas, A.Z.; Bhandi, S.H. Influence of Filler Composition on the Refractive Index of Four Different Enamel Shades of Composite Resins. *J. Contemp. Dent. Pract.* **2021**, *22*, 557–561.
43. Wang, X.J.; Milner, T.E.; de Boer, J.F.; Zhang, Y.; Pashley, D.H.; Nelson, J.S. Characterization of Dentin and Enamel by Use of Optical Coherence Tomography. *Appl. Opt.* **1999**, *38*, 2092–2096. [CrossRef]
44. Meng, Z.; Yao, X.S.; Yao, H.; Liang, Y.; Liu, T.; Li, Y.; Wang, G.; Lan, S. Measurement of the Refractive Index of Human Teeth by Optical Coherence Tomography. *J. Biomed. Opt.* **2009**, *14*, 034010. [CrossRef]
45. Heffernan, M.J.; Aquilino, S.A.; Diaz-Arnold, A.M.; Haselton, D.R.; Stanford, C.M.; Vargas, M.A. Relative Translucency of Six All-Ceramic Systems. Part II: Core and Veneer Materials. *J. Prosthet. Dent.* **2002**, *88*, 10–15. [CrossRef]
46. Oivanen, M.; Keulemans, F.; Garoushi, S.; Vallittu, P.K.; Lassila, L. The Effect of Refractive Index of Fillers and Polymer Matrix on Translucency and Color Matching of Dental Resin Composite. *Biomater. Investig. Dent.* **2021**, *8*, 48–53. [CrossRef]
47. Fujita, K.; Nishiyama, N.; Nemoto, K.; Okada, T.; Ikemi, T. Effect of Base Monomer's Refractive Index on Curing Depth and Polymerization Conversion of Photo-Cured Resin Composites. *Dent. Mater. J.* **2005**, *24*, 403–408. [CrossRef] [PubMed]
48. Son, S.-A.; Roh, H.-M.; Hur, B.; Kwon, Y.-H.; Park, J.-K. The Effect of Resin Thickness on Polymerization Characteristics of Silorane-Based Composite Resin. *Restor. Dent. Endod.* **2014**, *39*, 310–318. [CrossRef]
49. Arikawa, H.; Kanie, T.; Fujii, K.; Takahashi, H.; Ban, S. Effect of Filler Properties in Composite Resins on Light Transmittance Characteristics and Color. *Dent. Mater. J.* **2007**, *26*, 38–44. [CrossRef]
50. Howard, B.; Wilson, N.D.; Newman, S.M.; Pfeifer, C.S.; Stansbury, J.W. Relationships between Conversion, Temperature and Optical Properties during Composite Photopolymerization. *Acta Biomater.* **2010**, *6*, 2053–2059. [CrossRef]
51. Wee, A.G.; Lindsey, D.T.; Shroyer, K.M.; Johnston, W.M. Use of a Porcelain Color Discrimination Test to Evaluate Color Difference Formulas. *J. Prosthet. Dent.* **2007**, *98*, 101–109. [CrossRef]
52. Gómez-Polo, C.; Portillo Muñoz, M.; Lorenzo Luengo, M.C.; Vicente, P.; Galindo, P.; Martín Casado, A.M. Comparison of the CIELab and CIEDE2000 Color Difference Formulas. *J. Prosthet. Dent.* **2016**, *115*, 65–70. [CrossRef]
53. Gómez-Polo, C.; Montero, J.; Gómez-Polo, M.; Martin Casado, A. Comparison of the CIELab and CIEDE 2000 Color Difference Formulas on Gingival Color Space. *J. Prosthodont.* **2020**, *29*, 401–408. [CrossRef]
54. Ghinea, R.; Pérez, M.M.; Herrera, L.J.; Rivas, M.J.; Yebra, A.; Paravina, R.D. Color Difference Thresholds in Dental Ceramics. *J. Dent.* **2010**, *38* (Suppl. 2), e57–e64. [CrossRef]
55. Iyer, R.S.; Babani, V.R.; Yaman, P.; Dennison, J. Color Match Using Instrumental and Visual Methods for Single, Group, and Multi-Shade Composite Resins. *J. Esthet. Restor. Dent.* **2021**, *33*, 394–400. [CrossRef]
56. Islam, M.S.; Huda, N.; Mahendran, S.; Ac, S.A.; Nassar, M.; Rahman, M.M. The Blending Effect of Single-Shade Composite with Different Shades of Conventional Resin Composites—An In Vitro Study. *Eur. J. Dent.* **2023**, *17*, 342–348. [CrossRef]
57. Akgül, S.; Gündoğdu, C.; Bala, O. Effects of Storage Time and Restoration Depth on Instrumental Color Adjustment Potential of Universal Resin Composites. *J. Oral Sci.* **2022**, *64*, 49–52. [CrossRef] [PubMed]
58. Karabulut Gencer, B.; Acar, E.; Tarcın, B. Evaluation of Shade Matching in the Repair of Indirect Restorative Materials with Universal Shade Composites. *Eur. Oral Res.* **2023**, *57*, 41–48. [CrossRef] [PubMed]
59. Schneider, L.F.J.; Cavalcante, L.M.; Consani, S.; Ferracane, J.L. Effect of Co-Initiator Ratio on the Polymer Properties of Experimental Resin Composites Formulated with Camphorquinone and Phenyl-Propanedione. *Dent. Mater.* **2009**, *25*, 369–375. [CrossRef] [PubMed]

60. Wang, J.; Xu, C.; Nilsson, A.M.; Fernandes, D.L.A.; Niklasson, G.A. A Novel Phase Function Describing Light Scattering of Layers Containing Colloidal Nanospheres. *Nanoscale* **2019**, *11*, 7404–7413. [CrossRef]
61. Paolone, G.; Mandurino, M.; Scotti, N.; Cantatore, G.; Blatz, M.B. Color Stability of Bulk-Fill Compared to Conventional Resin-Based Composites: A Scoping Review. *J. Esthet. Restor. Dent.* **2023**, *35*, 657–676. [CrossRef]
62. Khayat, W.F. In Vitro Comparison of Optical Properties Between Single-Shade and Conventional Composite Resin Restorations. *Cureus* **2024**, *16*, e57664. [CrossRef]
63. Munoz, A.; Zhao, Z.; Paolone, G.; Louca, C.; Vichi, A. Flexural Strength of CAD/CAM Lithium-Based Silicate Glass-Ceramics: A Narrative Review. *Materials* **2023**, *16*, 4398. [CrossRef]

materials

MDPI

Article

Improving Bonding Durability in Dental Restorations: The Impact of Bioactive and Reinforcement Particles on Universal Adhesives

William Cunha Brandt [1], Isaías Donizeti Silva [1], Andreia Carneiro Matos [1], Flávia Gonçalves [1] and Leticia Boaro [2,*]

[1] Faculdade de Odontologia, Universidade Santo Amaro, Av. Prof. Eneas de Siqueira Neto, 340, São Paulo 04829-900, Brazil; williamcbrandt@yahoo.com.br (W.C.B.); isaiasdonizeti@gmail.com (I.D.S.); andreiacarneiro@gmail.com (A.C.M.); flgoncalves@prof.unisa.br (F.G.)

[2] College of Dentistry, University of Saskatchewan, 107 Wiggins Rd, Saskatoon, SK S7N 5E5, Canada

* Correspondence: leticiacidreiraboaro@gmail.com; Tel.: +1-(639)-318-3843

Abstract

Objective: This study aimed to evaluate the effect of incorporating bioactive particles (montmorillonite loaded with chlorhexidine, MMT/CHX) and different concentrations of silica nanoparticles (0%, 3%, 5%, 7%, 10%, and 15 wt%) into a universal dental adhesive on its degree of conversion, bond strength, water sorption, solubility, and antimicrobial activity. Materials and Methods: A universal adhesive was modified with 1 wt% MMT/CHX and varying amounts of silica nanoparticles. Degree of conversion was analyzed by Fourier transform infrared spectroscopy (FTIR), and microtensile bond strength was evaluated at 24 h, 6 months, and 12 months after water storage. Water sorption and solubility were measured according to ISO 4049, and antibacterial activity was tested against *Streptococcus mutans* using the agar diffusion method. Results: All experimental adhesives containing $\geq$7% silica showed significantly reduced water sorption and solubility. The presence of MMT/CHX imparted consistent antimicrobial activity across all experimental groups. Degree of conversion remained stable across all groups and storage periods. Notably, after 12 months, only the experimental groups maintained or improved bond strength, while the control group showed a significant reduction. Failure mode analysis indicated increased mechanical integrity with higher filler content. Conclusions: Incorporating 1 wt% MMT/CHX and $\geq$7 wt% silica into a universal adhesive improved long-term bond strength, reduced degradation, and introduced antibacterial properties without compromising polymer conversion. These findings support the potential of developing durable, bioactive adhesive systems for restorative dentistry. Clinical Significance: The incorporation of bioactive and reinforcing nanoparticles into universal adhesives enhances bond durability and introduces antibacterial properties without compromising polymerization. This innovation may lead to longer-lasting restorations and reduced risk of secondary caries in clinical practice.

Keywords: dental adhesive; bioactive particles; chlorhexidine; silica nanoparticles; bond strength; antimicrobial; degree of conversion; universal adhesive

1. Introduction

The advancement of adhesive dentistry has facilitated the development of more conservative restorative techniques, as well as the establishment of effective bonding between tooth structure and restoration [1–3]. To achieve this, three-step adhesive systems that utilize prior acid conditioning of dentin and enamel are considered the gold standard for ensuring adequate bonding of resin-based restorative materials to the dental substrate. According to various studies, this system provides high values of bond strength [4,5]. However, over time, the technique of acid conditioning of dentin can lead to increased permeability of the hybridized dentin, greater degradation of the bond, and, consequently, a reduction in bond strength [6]. This is primarily due to the activation of matrix metalloproteinases, which degrade dental collagen, thus impairing the tooth/restoration bond [7].

In order to reduce the activation of metalloproteinases that degrade the bond and also decrease clinical time for the fabrication of adhesive restorations, adhesive systems have been simplified. "Universal" single-bottle adhesives have been developed. In this adhesive system, the acid primer and adhesive resin are combined in a single bottle, reducing the adhesive application technique to one step [8,9].

Nonetheless, dental adhesives remain the weakest link in dental restorations, contributing to marginal gaps and consequently the development of secondary caries [10,11]. This limitation in bonding systems can lead to the need for restoration replacements and, therefore, the loss of healthy dental tissue. This problem may arise due to the low mechanical strength of adhesives when subjected to stress generated by polymerization shrinkage of composites, as well as the fragility of their polymeric structure, often porous due to the presence of hydrophilic components in their composition [12,13]. As such, in order to improve the durability of the adhesive interface and the mechanical properties of the adhesive interface, inorganic filler particles, ranging in size from 5 to 400 nm, were incorporated into the composition of these resinous materials [13–16]. These inorganic particles are added with the aim of reducing polymerization shrinkage, increasing cohesive strength, and enhancing the quality of the polymer formed, thereby promoting better sealing of the bonding interface [13,14].

The inorganic filler particles included in small proportions in dental adhesives need to penetrate the dentinal tubules to ensure uniform distribution of the filler particles throughout the adhesive layer and hybrid layer [15,16]. Therefore, it is necessary to incorporate nanometric-sized filler particles into these adhesive systems, with the subsequent possibility of integrating the inorganic particles throughout the entire extent of the applied adhesive resin. A previous study [14] showed that incorporating 10% by weight of 7 nm filler particles into hydrophobic resins of conventional three-step adhesive systems could improve the cohesive strength of this material without affecting the degree of conversion of the resinous polymer structure.

Another factor that may affect the tooth/restoration bond is the degradation of the adhesive bond. Both the adhesive polymer and the collagen present in the hybridized layer are susceptible to degradation. However, collagen degradation remains the primary concern [6]. Studies have shown that the prior application of chlorhexidine can neutralize the matrix metalloproteinases that degrade collagen. Therefore, the development of bioactive adhesives capable of neutralizing metalloproteinases would be of significant importance in increasing the longevity of dental restorations. Consequently, carrier particles such as nano-montmorillonite (MMT), which can release substances that inhibit metalloproteinases, such as chlorhexidine (CHX), may aid in this task [17,18]. This bioactive particle of MMT loaded with CHX has been previously described in the literature and showed promising results, especially in antibacterial activity in different polymeric matrices such as di-methacrylate [17], poly methyl-methacrylate [18], and epoxy resin [19], but is still not being tested in dental adhesive systems.

New formulations of simplified dental adhesives (single-bottle systems), containing varying amounts of nanometric filler particles, are important for evaluating the development of bonding agents with improved physicomechanical properties [20]. Thus, it becomes essential to assess the effect of incorporating different quantities of nanometric inorganic particles and bioactive particles into universal adhesives on the degree of conversion and bond strength, and to analyze the feasibility of developing bioactive adhesives.

Building on the concepts outlined above, the development of a bioactive adhesive system capable of controlled chlorhexidine (CHX) release, reinforced with an increased concentration of filler, holds significant promise for creating durable, long-lasting restorations. This approach not only enhances the adhesive mechanical properties but also offers antibacterial benefits, potentially improving the longevity and performance of dental restorations in the oral environment.

Therefore, the purpose of this study was to analyze (1) the addition of a bioactive particle (MMT/CHX) and (2) the different concentrations of silica nanoparticle (0%, 3%, 5%, 7%, 10%, and 15 wt%) on the degree of conversion and bond strength of a universal adhesive with bioactive properties after 24 h, 6 months, and 12 months of storage.

The null hypothesis is that the incorporation of both particles (silica and MMT/CHX) will not affect the evaluated properties independently of the storage period.

2. Materials and Methods

The commercially available universal self-etching adhesive YBond Universal (Yller Biomaterials, Neodent, Pelotas, Brazil) base was used as the standard matrix. According to the manufacturer, its polymeric matrix is composed by hydrophilic methacrylates monomers, hydrophobic methacrylates monomers, initiators, stabilizers, and silane, and it has water and ethanol as solvent. The experimental groups are described in Figure 1. The control group (C) did not receive any particles. The bioactive groups (B-B15) received 1% in weight of MMT/CHX particles. The MMT/CHX particles were synthesized as described before [17–19], then briefly CHX was first incorporated into the MMT nanoparticles by dispersing them in an aqueous solution of CHX at a 10% weight-to-weight ratio (*w*/*w*). The mixture was continuously stirred for 3 h at a temperature of 80 °C. Following this emulsion process, the compound was freeze-dried for approximately 6 h. Following this process, the resulting MMT/CHX particles contain 7 wt% of CHX intercalated within their lamellar structure. Different amounts of nanosized silica particles (7 nm, Aerosil 320, Degussa, Germany) were added to the bioactive adhesive by the manufacturer and 1 wt% MMT/CHX particles were added using a mechanical mixer (SpeedMixer DAC 150 FVZ, Hauschild, Farmington Hills, MI, USA) at 2500 rpm for 30 s at 21 °C. Around 10 mL of each adhesive was prepared. No filler agglomeration was visually detected in the samples. All samples were activated using the BluePhase LED light source (Ivoclar Vivadent, Schaan, Liechtenstein).

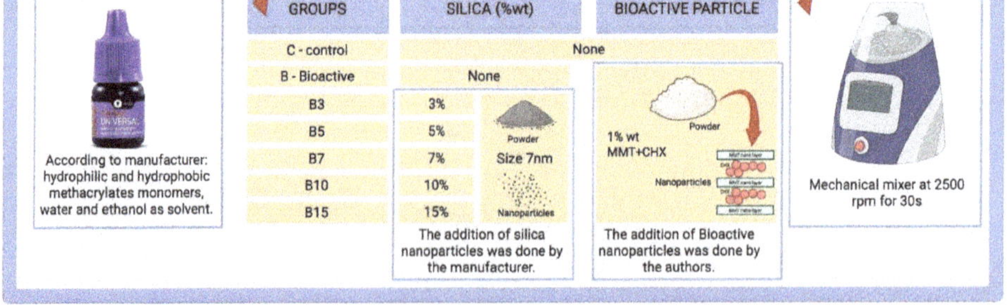

Figure 1. Experimental groups and filler addition. Created in BioRender. Boaro, L. (2025) https://BioRender.com/i62y660 (accessed on 7 September 2025) (Agreement number: ET28QNL37C).

2.1. Sorption and Solubility

Sorption and solubility were determined according to ISO 4049 standards [21]. Cylindrical specimens with a diameter of 15 mm and a height of 1 mm were fabricated using a steel mold (n = 5). Photoactivation was performed with a dose of 18 J/cm^2 (20 s) in each side. A single exposure was able to cover the entire diameter of the samples.

The specimens were then subjected to desiccation in a vacuum desiccator at 37 °C for 14 days. The specimens were weighed on an analytical balance to obtain m_1. The diameter and height of each specimen were measured to calculate the volume. The specimens were immersed in distilled water at 37 °C for seven days, lightly dried with absorbent paper, and weighed again to obtain m_2. They were then desiccated as previously described for 14 days and weighed to obtain m_3. Sorption and solubility were calculated for each specimen using the following formulas:

$$SR = \frac{m2 - m1}{V} \quad SL = \frac{m1 - m3}{V}$$

where SR is sorption; SL is solubility; m1 is the mass after the initial drying of the specimen (μg); m2 is the mass after the immersion period in water (μg); m3 is the final mass after desiccation (μg); V is the specimen volume (mm^3).

2.2. Bacterial Sensitivity Test by Agar Diffusion Technique (Inhibition Halo)

Disc specimens with 5 mm in diameter and 1 mm in height were made using a silicone mold and photoactivation was performed with a dose of 18 J/cm^2 (20 s). The agar diffusion technique was performed following the recommendations of the CLSI—Clinical and Laboratory Standards Institute (Performance Standards for Antimicrobial Disk Susceptibility Tests: Approved Standard—Eighth Edition, M02-A12) [22]. A bacterial suspension of *Streptococcus mutans* UA159 was adjusted in a spectrophotometer with an absorbance of 0.1 at 660 nm, which is equivalent to 1–2 × 10^8 CFU/mL. A sterile swab was immersed in this solution and sprayed in a BHI culture plate. Five samples of each material (n = 5) were placed on the surface of the seeded plate and incubated in anaerobic conditions at 37 °C for 24 h. The inhibition halo was measured using a digital caliper, in two perpendicular directions. The mean of these measurements was considered the inhibition halo diameter. The samples' diameters were also measured in order to avoid that small variation in sample diameter affects the result.

2.3. Degree of Conversion

For each group (n = 10), bar shape specimens (7 mm length × 2 mm width × 1 mm thickness) were made using a silicon mold. The degree of conversion was evaluated by Fourier Transform Infrared Spectroscopy (mid-FTIR, Spectrum 100—PerkinElmer, Shelton, CT, USA), with a coupled attenuated total reflectance element—ATR, which has a horizontal Zinc Selenide crystal (Pike Technologies, Madison, WI, USA) in the center that functions as an active substrate for infrared rays. For the measurement, an unpolymerized drop of the experimental adhesive was initially placed on the zinc selenide crystal of the FTIR device, and then the polymerized specimens were positioned one at a time for the reading. Spectra were obtained before (unpolymerized) 24 h, 6 months, and 12 months after photoactivation with co-addition of 16 scans and a resolution of 4 cm^{-1}. The polymerization reaction occurred by the breaking of aliphatic double carbon bonds of dimethacrylates monomers, so the corresponding area under 1638 cm^{-1} was used to calculate the degree of conversion. Also, the absorption band area under the 1608 cm^{-1}, corresponding to aromatic double carbon of 2,2-bis [4-[2-hydroxy-3-methacryloxy) propoxi]phenyl]-propane, was used as internal standard in the calculus, since it is not affected by polymerization reactions [23], for uncured and cured materials.

2.4. Bond Strength

This study was previously submitted and approved by the Research Ethics Committee (CAAE #4,989,582). A total of 210 pristine human molar teeth extracted for therapeutic reasons were selected. Teeth were randomly distributed into the groups ($n = 10$) considering 7 groups of experimental adhesives and 3 different storage periods (24 h, 6 months, and 12 months). Each tooth was sectioned twice according to the method shown in Figure 2, using diamond discs under constant water cooling. The occlusal dentin surface was abraded using silicon carbide sandpaper (#220, 400, and 600) to obtain flat surfaces of medium dentin, and also to simulate a newly formed smear-layer. The experimental adhesives (Figure 1) were actively applied for 20 s, the solvent was evaporated with an air jet, and another layer was applied repeating the same protocol, then photoactivated with a dose of 18 J/cm^2 (20 s). The restoration was conducted using a composite (Filtek Z350, 3M ESPE, shade A1) with 6 mm in diameter and a thickness of 2 mm using a silicone matrix. Then, a polyester strip was positioned on top of the restoration with the silicon matrix and a 500 g weight was placed on the strip. After 10 s, the weight was removed, and the composite was photoactivated with a dose of 18 J/cm^2 (20 s). The restored teeth were then stored in water and in a dark environment at 37 °C for 24 h. After this period, the teeth were sectioned in bar shaped specimens with 1 × 1 mm, resulting in an adhesive area of approximately 1 mm^2. The dimensions of each specimen were measured using a digital caliper to individualize the cross-sectioned area and to use in the bond strength calculus. At least 10 specimens of each tooth were individually stored, and tested in 24 h, 6 months, and 12 months (Figure 2). The microtensile test was performed using a universal testing machine (EMIC DL500, São José dos Pinhais, Brazil) at a speed of 0.5 mm/min. The bond strength was calculated by dividing the maximum load (N) required for failure by the area verified for each specimen and expressed in MPa.

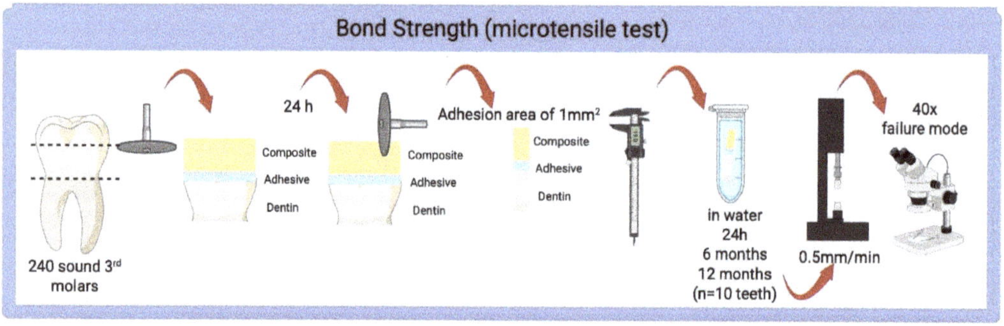

Figure 2. Experimental design for the bond strength. Created in BioRender. Boaro, L. (2025) https://BioRender.com/i62y660 (accessed on 7 September 2025) (Agreement number: ET28QNL37C).

2.5. Failure Mode

To analyze the failure mode, the samples were analyzed using an optical microscope at 40× magnification and classified as adhesive, cohesive (in dentin or composite resin), or mixed (combination of adhesive and cohesive).

2.6. Statistical Analyses

Data from the sorption, solubility, and inhibition halo were analyzed using a one-way ANOVA/Tukey's test ($p < 0.05$). Data from degree of conversion and bond strength were analyzed using a two-way ANOVA/Tukey's test ($p < 0.05$) (factors group and storage period).

3. Results

The addition of 7% colloidal silica filler or more was able to significantly decrease the sorption and the solubility of the experimental adhesives in relation to the control group (Table 1, Figures S1 and S2).

Table 1. Parameter of sorption and solubility (μg/mm^3) for control and bioactive dental adhesives (mean and standard deviation). The letters indicate statistical comparisons among mean. In the same column, values followed by the same letter do not present statistical differences ($p > 0.05$).

Group	Sorption (μg/mm^3)	Solubility (μg/mm^3)
C—Control	327 (34) a	130 (17) a
B—Bioactive	262 (25) ab	97 (11) ab
B3	270 (23) ab	98 (10) ab
B5	272 (59) ab	100 (26) ab
B7	235 (36) b	88 (17) b
B10	226 (42) b	83 (17) b
B15	220 (17) b	84 (8) b

The presence of 1% MMT/chlorhexidine in all the bioactive materials was able to present the inhibition halo against *S. mutans* independently of the silica concentration. In contrast, the control group, with the absence of MTT/chlorhexidine particles, was not able to generate an inhibition halo against the *S. mutans* (Figure 3).

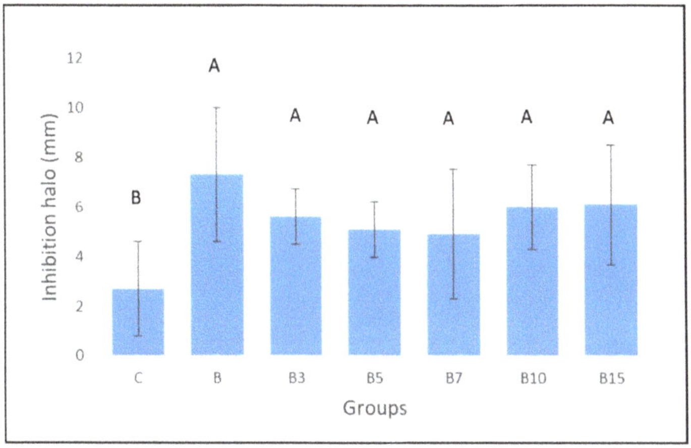

Figure 3. Means and standard deviation of inhibition halo (mm). The letters indicate statistical comparisons among mean. Values followed by the same letter do not present statistical differences ($p > 0.05$).

There is no significant difference in the degree of conversion (DC) of the materials studied at 6 or 12 months (Table 2 and Figure S3). Also, there is no difference between conversion of one material after 24 h and 6 months or 12 months. The only exception is the material with 3% colloidal silica, which presented lower conversion than the material with 7% colloidal silica at 24 h and also presented an increase of conversion from 24 h to 6 months.

Table 2. Degree of conversion (%) for control and bioactive dental adhesives at 6 and 12 months (mean and standard deviation). The letters indicate statistical comparisons among mean. In the same column, values followed by the same lowercase letter do not present statistical differences ($p > 0.05$). In the same row, values followed by the same uppercase letter do not present statistical differences ($p > 0.05$).

Group	Degree of Conversion %		
	24 h	**6 Months**	**12 Months**
C—Control	87 (3) abA	89 (3) aA	88 (2) aA
B—Bioactive	70 (7) bA	89 (7) aA	87 (5) aA
B3	69 (2) bB	93 (1) aA	92 (3) aA
B5	85 (10) abA	91 (10) aA	92 (7) aA
B7	93 (10) aA	96 (6) aA	94 (7) aA
B10	91 (14) aA	99 (12) aA	91 (4) aA
B15	70 (4) bA	88 (7) aA	88 (6) aA

The bond strength was similar among all the experimental and control materials after 24 h and 6 months. However, after 12 months the bond strength was higher for all experimental materials in relation to the control. In addition, all the experimental materials were able to maintain the bond strength values along the 12 months except the control materials, which presented a decrease in this property after 12 months (Table 3, Figure S4).

Table 3. Bond Strength (MPa) for control and bioactive dental adhesives at 6 and 12 months (mean and standard deviation). The letters indicate statistical comparisons among mean. In the same column, values followed by the same lowercase letter do not present statistical differences ($p > 0.05$). In the same row, values followed by the same uppercase letter do not present statistical differences ($p > 0.05$).

Group	Bond Strength (MPa)		
	24 h	**6 Months**	**12 Months**
C—Control	12 (4) aA	9 (2) aA	6 (4) bB
B—Bioactive	10 (3) aA	9 (4) aA	8 (3) aA
B3	9 (3) aA	10 (3) aA	9 (4) aA
B5	11 (2) aA	10 (2) aA	9 (4) aA
B7	13 (3) aA	9 (3) aA	8 (3) aA
B10	12 (4) aA	10 (3) aA	9 (5) aA
B15	9 (3) aA	10 (4) aA	9 (3) aA

The correlation analysis among the bond strength at 12 months and sorption and solubility data are presented in Figure 4. There can be observed a moderate correlation of bond strength with sorption ($R^2 = 0.56$) and with solubility ($R^2 = 0.69$).

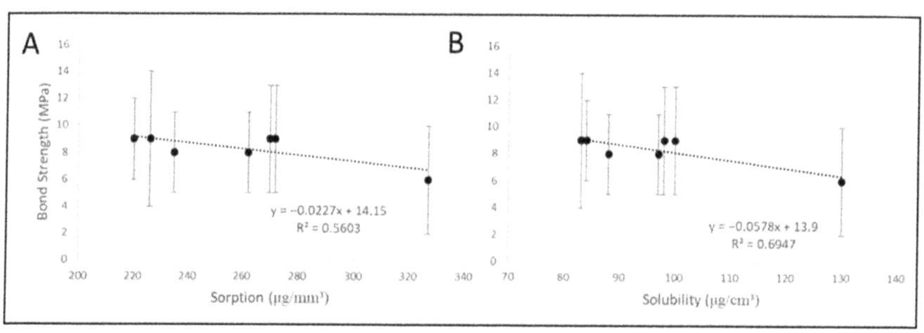

Figure 4. Correlation analysis between (**A**) bond strength at 12 months (MPa) and sorption (µg/mm^3) of control and bioactive adhesives, and (**B**) bond strength at 12 months (MPa) and solubility (µg/mm^3).

When observing the failure mode of the samples in the bond strength test, the cohesive failures are only observed for the control materials and materials with lower filler concentration (B1 to B5) independently of the storage time.

The storage time affected the failure mode (Figure 5). At 24 h the majority of failures were adhesive while at 6 and 12 months the mixed failures were predominant. The difference between the percentage of adhesive and mixed failures is also affected by filler concentration, since the differences are more accentuated in materials with a higher filler amount, independently of the storage time.

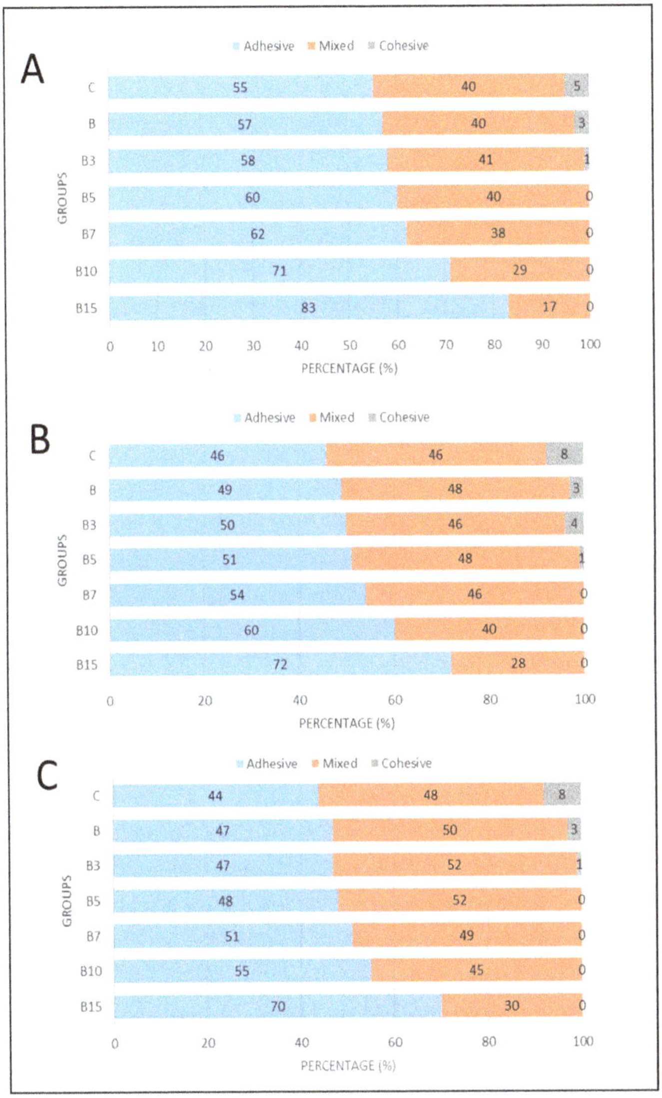

Figure 5. Percentage of adhesive, mixed, or cohesive failure mode after different lengths of time in storage. (**A**) 24 h of storage, (**B**) 6 months of storage, and (**C**) 12 months of storage.

4. Discussion

In the present study, it was demonstrated that the experimental adhesives suggested were not only able to maintain the bond strength along 12 months, in contrast to the control material, but also presented antimicrobial activity against *S. mutans* without jeopardizing the conversion of the material. Furthermore, the addition of 1 wt% MMT/CHX and 7 wt% colloidal filler or more into the adhesives decreased the water sorption and solubility. So, the null hypothesis that the incorporation of both particles (silica and MMT/CHX) will not affect the evaluated properties independently of the storage period was rejected.

Out of all the adhesives evaluated, only control and experimental were able to maintain the bond strength after 6 months of storage, but only the experimental materials were able to maintain the bond strength after 12 months of storage. In fact, it has been shown that commercial materials present a reduction in bond strength depending on the time [24,25], and it occurs due to two main factors: the degradation of the adhesive layer by the enzymatic action of metalloproteinases [26,27] and by the hydrolytic degradation [27,28]. The experimental adhesives tested acted in both of these factors. It is known that the presence of chlorhexidine is able to inhibit the action of metalloproteinases enzymes [29,30], and apparently the concentration of 1 wt% was satisfactory to this purpose. In addition, the incorporation of filler particles from 7 to 15% significantly decreased the sorption and solubility of the materials, resulting in a decrease in hydrolytic degradation. The correlation analysis among the variables confirms these hypotheses, showing moderated inverse correlations between bond strength and sorption, and also between bond strength and solubility (Figure 3). These results are in agreement with other studies, which observe reduction in hydrolytic degradation in function of the filler amount [27,28].

The failure pattern indicated that increased SiO_2 filler content enhanced the mechanical properties of the adhesive, leading to fewer mixed and cohesive failures in initial tests (24 h). However, after 6 and 12 months, a general increase in mixed and cohesive failures was noted in all the materials, likely due to degradation in aqueous media, which was able to reduce the adhesive's mechanical properties over time, even though it did not significantly affect the bond strength. Similar results were observed when PMAA-grafted nanoclay was added in dental adhesives, enhancing microshear bond strength with even small amounts of nanoclay [31].

Another important aspect of the experimental adhesive evaluated is that all presented similar conversion to the control group. Once the degree of conversion is related to cytotoxicity and some mechanical properties [32], the maintenance of the conversion can suggest similar performance. In fact, a related study demonstrated that the inclusion of MMT nanoclays enabled the production of dental composites with low cytotoxicity and reduced polymerization shrinkage [33], without compromising essential physical–mechanical properties like flexural strength, modulus of elasticity, water sorption, water solubility, and hygroscopic behavior. Similarly, it has been reported that resins with MMT/CHX particles exhibited similar conversion to control material without the particles in dental composites and acrylic resin, suggesting that the low filler content had little impact on the polymerization process [34]. In agreement, some authors have demonstrated that particles with size higher than the light wavelength do not interfere in the light scattering and can maintain the material conversion [35].

Finally, it should be highlighted that the presence of 1 wt% MTT/CHX particles guarantees an antimicrobial effect against *S. mutans* in all experimental adhesives, which is an advantage in reducing biofilm growth and can possibly make difficult the development of secondary decay. The antimicrobial effect of MMT/CHX has been observed in previous studies [20,21], either in immediate or late effect [19,36] being observed along 12 months, when added at 5 wt% in dental composites [36].

5. Conclusions

According to the limitation of the present in vitro study, regarding the evaluation of only one polymeric matrix and one MMT/CHX concentration, and the absence of mechanical load along the storage, it can be concluded that the addition of 1 wt% MMT/CHX and 7 wt% colloidal silica or more was able to maintain the bond strength of experimental adhesives along 12 months, decrease the water sorption and solubility of materials, and also present antimicrobial activity against *S. mutans*.

Supplementary Materials: The following supporting information can be downloaded at: https://www.mdpi.com/article/10.3390/ma18194433/s1, Figure S1: Mean and standard deviation of sorption (µg/mm^3) of the experimental and control materials; Figure S2: Mean and standard deviation of solubility (µg/mm^3) of the experimental and control materials; Figure S3: Mean and standard deviation of degree of conversion (%) of the experimental and control materials measured at 24 h, 6 and 12 months; Figure S4: Mean and standard deviation of degree of conversion (%) of the experimental and control materials measured at 24 h, 6 and 12 months. (*) indicates the only material that is statically different from the others after 12 months of storage.

Author Contributions: The conception and design of this study—W.C.B. and L.B.; acquisition of data—I.D.S., A.C.M. and F.G.; analysis and interpretation of data—F.G., W.C.B. and L.B.; drafting the article—I.D.S., A.C.M. and F.G.; revising it critically for important intellectual content—W.C.B., F.G. and L.B.; final approval of the version to be submitted—all the authors; project supervision and funding raising—L.B. All authors have read and agreed to the published version of the manuscript.

Funding: This research was funded by the São Paulo Research Foundation (FAPESP), Brazil. Process number 2016/01319-9. And The APC was funded by University of Saskatchewan College of Dentistry Startup fund. The funders had no role in study design, data collection and analysis, decision to publish, or preparation of the manuscript.

Institutional Review Board Statement: The study was conducted in accordance with the Declaration of Helsinki, and approved by the Ethics Committee of Universidade Santo Amaro (CAAE: 46805121.4.0000.0081; protocol code 4.989.582 and 22 September 2021).

Informed Consent Statement: Informed consent was obtained from all subjects involved in the study.

Data Availability Statement: The original contributions presented in this study are included in the article. Further inquiries can be directed to the corresponding author.

Conflicts of Interest: The authors declare no conflict of interest.

References

1. Isolan, C.P.; Sarkis-Onofre, R.; Lima, G.S.; Moraes, R.R. Bonding to Sound and Caries-Affected Dentin: A Systematic Review and Meta-Analysis. *J. Adhes. Dent.* **2018**, *20*, 7–18. [CrossRef]
2. Borges, B.C.; Souza-Junior, E.J.; Brandt, W.C.; Loguercio, A.D.; Montes, M.A.; Puppin-Rontani, R.M.; Sinhoreti, M.A.C. Degree of conversion of simplified contemporary adhesive systems as influenced by extended air-activated or passive solvent volatilization modes. *Oper. Dent.* **2012**, *37*, 246–252. [CrossRef] [PubMed]
3. Saini, R.S.; Vyas, R.; Vaddamanu, S.K.; Quadri, S.A.; Mosaddad, S.A.; Heboyan, A. Efficacy of different adhesive systems in bonding direct resin composite restorations: A systematic review and meta-analysis. *Evid.-Based Dent.* **2025**, *26*, 115. [CrossRef] [PubMed]
4. Perdigão, J.; Lopes, M.M.; Gomes, G. In vitro bonding performance of self-etch adhesives: II--ultramorphological evaluation. *Oper. Dent.* **2008**, *33*, 534–549. [CrossRef] [PubMed]
5. Brackett, W.W.; Haisch, L.D.; Pearce, M.G.; Brackett, M.G. Microleakage of Class V resin composite restorations placed with self-etching adhesives. *J. Prosthet. Dent.* **2004**, *91*, 42–45. [CrossRef]

6. Mazzoni, A.; Angeloni, V.; Comba, A.; Maravic, T.; Cadenaro, M.; Tezvergil-Mutluay, A.; Pashley, D.H.; Tay, F.R.; Breschi, L. Cross-linking effect on dentin bond strength and MMPs activity. *Dent. Mater.* **2018**, *34*, 288–295. [CrossRef]
7. Sinha, D.J.; Jaiswal, N.; Vasudeva, A.; Garg, P.; Tyagi, S.P.; Chandra, P. Comparative evaluation of the effect of chlorhexidine and Aloe barbadensis Miller (*Aloe vera*) on dentin stabilization using shear bond testing. *J. Conserv. Dent.* **2016**, *19*, 406–409. [CrossRef]
8. Pashley, D.H.; Tay, F.R.; Breschi, L.; Tjäderhane, L.; Carvalho, R.M.; Carrilho, M.; Tezvergil-Mutluay, A. State of the art etch-and-rinse adhesives. *Dent. Mater.* **2011**, *27*, 1–16. [CrossRef]
9. Brkanović, S.; Sever, E.K.; Vukelja, J.; Ivica, A.; Miletić, I.; Krmek, S.J. Comparison of Different Universal Adhesive Systems on Dentin Bond Strength. *Materials* **2023**, *16*, 1530. [CrossRef]
10. Kemp-Scholte, C.M.; Davidson, C.L. Complete marginal seal of Class V resin composite restorations effected by increased flexibility. *J. Dent. Res.* **1990**, *69*, 1240–1243. [CrossRef]
11. Hashimoto, M.; Ohno, H.; Sano, H.; Kaga, M.; Oguchi, H. Degradation patterns of different adhesives and bonding procedures. *J. Biomed. Mater. Res. B Appl. Biomater.* **2003**, *66*, 324–330. [CrossRef] [PubMed]
12. Sano, H.; Takatsu, T.; Ciucchi, B.; Russell, C.M.; Pashley, D.H. Tensile properties of resin-infiltrated demineralized human dentin. *J. Dent. Res.* **1995**, *74*, 1093–1102. [CrossRef] [PubMed]
13. Van Landuyt, K.L.; Snauwaert, J.; De Munck, J.; Peumans, M.; Yoshida, Y.; Poitevin, A.; Coutinho, E.; Suzuki, K.; Lambrechts, P.; Van Meerbeek, B. Systematic review of the chemical composition of contemporary dental adhesives. *Biomaterials* **2007**, *28*, 3757–3785. [CrossRef] [PubMed]
14. Conde, M.C.; Zanchi, C.H.; Rodrigues-Junior, S.A.; Carreño, N.L.; Ogliari, F.A.; Piva, E. Nanofiller loading level: Influence on selected properties of an adhesive resin. *J. Dent.* **2009**, *37*, 331–335. [CrossRef]
15. Giannini, M.; Mettenburg, D.; Arrais, C.A.; Rueggeberg, F.A. The effect of filler addition on biaxial flexure strength and modulus of commercial dentin bonding systems. *Quintessence Int.* **2011**, *42*, e39–e43.
16. Sharan, J.; Singh, S.; Lale, S.V.; Mishra, M.; Koul, V.; Kharbanda, P. Applications of Nanomaterials in Dental Science: A Review. *J. Nanosci. Nanotechnol.* **2017**, *17*, 2235–2255. [CrossRef]
17. Boaro, L.C.C.; Campos, L.M.; Varca, G.H.C.; Dos Santos, T.M.R.; Marques, P.A.; Sugii, M.M.; Saldanha, N.R.; Cogo-Müller, K.; Brandt, W.C.; Braga, R.R.; et al. Antibacterial resin-based composite containing chlorhexidine for dental applications. *Dent. Mater.* **2019**, *35*, 909–918. [CrossRef]
18. Moffa, E.B.; Malheiros, S.S.; Silva, L.T.S.; Branco, D.I.; Grassia Junior, R.C.F.; Brandt, W.C.; Goncalves, F.; Barao, V.A.R.; Boaro, L.C.C. Antimicrobial activity of PMMA enriched with nano-clay loaded with metronidazole and chlorhexidine. *Braz. Oral Res.* **2024**, *38*, e110. [CrossRef]
19. Gonçalves, F.; Campos, L.M.d.P.; Sanches, L.K.F.; Silva, L.T.S.; Santos, T.M.R.d.; Varca, G.H.C.; Lopes, D.P.; Cogo-Muller, K.; Parra, D.F.; Braga, R.R.; et al. Antimicrobial activity and physicochemical performance of a modified endodontic sealer. *Res. Soc. Dev.* **2020**, *9*, e069119401. [CrossRef]
20. da Silva, T.S.P.; de Castro, R.F.; Magno, M.B.; Maia, L.C.; Silva e Souza, M.H.d. Do HEMA-free adhesive systems have better clinical performance than HEMA-containing systems in noncarious cervical lesions? A systematic review and meta-analysis. *J. Dent.* **2018**, *74*, 1–14. [CrossRef]
21. *ISO 4049:2019*; Dentistry—Polymer-Based Restorative Materials. International Organization for Standardization: Geneva, Switzerland, 2019.
22. CLSI—Clinical and Laboratory Standards Institute. *Performance Standards for Antimicrobial Disk Susceptibility Tests: Approved Standard—Twelfth Edition (M02-A12)*; Clinical and Laboratory Standards Institute: Wayne, PA, USA, 2015.
23. Rueggeberg, F.A.; Hashinger, D.T.; Fairhurst, C.W. Calibration of FTIR conversion analysis of contemporary dental resin composites. *Dent. Mater.* **1990**, *6*, 241–249. [CrossRef] [PubMed]
24. Karadas, M.; Bedir, F.; Demirbuga, S. The role of etching protocols on bond strength of universal adhesives applied to caries affected dentin: A systematic review and meta-analysis. *Clin. Oral Investig.* **2024**, *28*, 683. [CrossRef] [PubMed]
25. Angelo, E.; Guerra, A.; Vitti, R.; Martins, L.R.M. The Effect of Ethanol Associated with Universal Adhesive on Resin Composite Adhesion to Different Dentin Depths: A Long-Term In Vitro Study. *Eur. J. Prosthodont. Restor. Dent.* **2023**, *31*, 254–261. [PubMed]
26. Lewis, N.V.; Aggarwal, S.; Borse, N.N.; Sonawane, S.; Dhatavkar, P.; Digholkar, R.; Agarwal, D. The Effect of Matrix Metalloproteinase Inhibitors on the Microtensile Bond Strength of Dentin Bonding Agents in Caries Affected Dentin: A Systematic Review. *J. Int. Soc. Prev. Community Dent.* **2023**, *13*, 173–184. [CrossRef]
27. Mokeem, L.S.; Garcia, I.M.; Melo, M.A. Degradation and Failure Phenomena at the Dentin Bonding Interface. *Biomedicines* **2023**, *11*, 1256. [CrossRef]
28. Mocharko, V.; Mascarenhas, P.; Azul, A.M.; Delgado, A.H.S. In Search of Novel Degradation-Resistant Monomers for Adhesive Dentistry: A Systematic Review and Meta-Analysis. *Biomedicines* **2022**, *10*, 3104. [CrossRef]

29. Narayanan, S.K.; Hari, K.; Mathew, J.; Sukumaran, A.; Joy, B.; Mathew, J. Effect of MMP Inhibitors on Shear Bond Strength of Adhesive to Dentin after Different Drying Techniques: An In-Vitro Study. *J. Pharm. Bioallied Sci.* **2024**, *16* (Suppl. S5), S4639–S4642. [CrossRef]
30. Stanislawczuk, R.; Reis, A.; Loguercio, A.D. A 2-year in vitro evaluation of a chlorhexidine-containing acid on the durability of resin-dentin interfaces. *J. Dent.* **2011**, *39*, 40–47. [CrossRef]
31. Solhi, L.; Atai, M.; Nodehi, A.; Imani, M. A novel dentin bonding system containing poly(methacrylic acid) grafted nanoclay: Synthesis, characterization and properties. *Dent. Mater.* **2012**, *28*, 1041–1050. [CrossRef]
32. Silva, I.D.; Boaro, L.C.C.; Muniz, B.V.; Cogo-Muller, K.; Gonçalves, F.; Brandt, W.C. The impact of chitosan in experimental resin with different photoinitiator systems. *J. Mech. Behav. Biomed. Mater.* **2024**, *150*, 106323. [CrossRef]
33. Ritto, F.P.; da Silva, E.M.; Borges, A.L.S.; Borges, M.A.P.; Sampaio-Filho, H.R. Fabrication and characterization of low-shrinkage dental composites containing montmorillonite nanoclay. *Odontology* **2022**, *110*, 35–43. [CrossRef]
34. Encalada-Alayola, J.J.; Veranes-Pantoja, Y.; Uribe-Calderón, J.A.; Cauich-Rodríguez, J.V.; Cervantes-Uc, J.M. Effect of Type and Concentration of Nanoclay on the Mechanical and Physicochemical Properties of Bis-GMA/TTEGDMA Dental Resins. *Polymers* **2020**, *12*, 601. [CrossRef]
35. Halvorson, R.H.; Erickson, R.L.; Davidson, C.L. The effect of filler and silane content on conversion of resin-based composite. *Dent. Mater.* **2003**, *19*, 327–333. [CrossRef]
36. Gonçalves, F.; Silva, L.S.T.; Roschel, J.N.; Souza, G.; Campos, L.M.; Varca, G.; Parra, D.; Perez, M.A.; Gordilho, A.C.; Brandt, W.C.; et al. Antibacterial resin composite with sustained chlorhexidine release—one-year in vitro study. *Pharmaceutics* **2025**, *17*, 1144. [CrossRef]

materials

MDPI

Article

Implants Placed with a Ring Technique Using Inlay and Onlay Block Xenografts in the Mandible of Rabbits

Naoki Kaneko [1], Samuel Porfirio Xavier [2], Kenzo Morinaga [1], Daniele Botticelli [1,3,*], Erick Ricardo Silva [2], Yasushi Nakajima [1,2] and Shunsuke Baba [1]

1 Department of Oral Implantology, Osaka Dental University, 8-1 Kuzuhahanazonocho, Hirakata 573-1121, Osaka, Japan; dentalkei@outlook.jp (N.K.); morinaga-k@cc.osaka-dent.ac.jp (K.M.); y.nakajima@me.com (Y.N.); baba-s@cc.osaka-dent.ac.jp (S.B.)
2 Department of Oral and Maxillofacial Surgery and Periodontology, Faculty of Dentistry of Ribeirão Preto, University of São Paulo, Av. do Café-Subsetor Oeste-11 (N-11), Ribeirão Preto 14040-904, SP, Brazil; spx@forp.usp.br (S.P.X.); erickricardo.rp@gmail.com (E.R.S.)
3 ARDEC Academy, 47923 Rimini, Italy
* Correspondence: daniele.botticelli@gmail.com

Abstract: Background: Xenogenous bone has been proposed as an alternative to overcome the disadvantages of autogenous grafting. The aim of the present study was to study bone dynamics at inlay and onlay xenografts used for bone augmentation applying a ring technique. Methods: The bone at the lateral surface of the mandibular angle of 12 adult male New Zealand White rabbits was exposed bilaterally. The cortical layer received multiple perforations on one side of the mandible, and a xenograft block of collagenated cancellous equine bone, 7 mm in diameter and 3 mm in width, was fixed on the prepared surface using an implant (onlay group). On the opposite side, a defect 7 mm in diameter and 3 mm in depth was prepared, and the xenograft block was adapted to the defect and fixed with an implant (inlay group). Results: After ten weeks of healing, in the onlay grafts, new bone was mainly formed on the trabeculae surface, reaching in some specimens the most coronal regions of the block. In the inlay grafts, new bone was found arranged on the trabecular surfaces but also occupying the spaces among the trabeculae. The entrance of the defect was often found close to the top of the block by newly formed bone. A higher percentage of new bone was found in the inlay (19.0 ± 9.3%) compared to the onlay (10.4 ± 7.4%) groups ($p = 0.031$). The mean gain in osseointegration at the implant in relation to the base of the original 3 mm deep defect was 0.95 ± 1.05% in the onlay group and 0.78 ± 0.71% in the inlay group ($p = 0.603$). Conclusion: The inlay grafts exhibited a higher new bone percentage than the onlay block grafts possibly due to the defect conformation that presented more sources for bone growth. The trabecular conformation and the composition of the grafts made possible the expression of the osteoconductive properties of the material used. This resulted, in several specimens, in the growth of bone on the graft trabeculae toward the most superior regions in both groups and in the closure of the coronal entrance of the defects in the inlay group. The clinical relevance of this experiment is that the ring technique applied as an inlay method could be suitable for bone augmentation.

Keywords: animal study; bone healing; histology; lateral augmentation; bone transplantation; biomaterial; bone defect; inlay; onlay; xenograft

1. Introduction

An atrophied posterior mandible, because of tooth loss, periodontal pathologies, tumor removal, trauma, or congenital diseases, represents a challenge for implant-supported rehabilitation because of the reduction in bone volume between the residual alveolar ridge and the mandibular canal [1–3]. Bone augmentation has become an essential component of implant dentistry in this scenario [4–6].

The inlay technique has proven to be highly effective for the incorporation of bone grafts, with low resorption over time and high implant survival and success rates [7–9]. Although good results have been reported for posterior mandibular bone augmentation using this technique [10–13], it demands considerable surgical experience, and at least 4 to 6 mm of bone height over the mandibular canal is needed [11,12].

Onlay bone grafts have been successfully used in mandibular bone augmentation. This technique has been associated with high rates of bone resorption before implant placement [2,14]. The soft tissue quality is the primary consideration during the reconstruction of the posterior mandibular region. A lack of keratinized tissue may contribute to wound dehiscence, infection, and subsequent necrosis of the graft [15].

Autogenous bone harvested from either extra- or intraoral donor sites is the gold-standard graft for alveolar ridge augmentation because of its osteoconductive, osteoinductive, and osteogenic properties [16–19]. Nevertheless, autografts have several disadvantages related to complications at the donor site, limitation of bone surgical morbidity at the donor site, postoperative pain, limited bone disposal, increased surgical time, and financial costs [20–25].

To address the drawbacks of autologous grafting, xenogenous bone has been proposed as an alternative [26–28]. Using xenogenous bone blocks from both equine and autogenic sources for onlay mandibular augmentation in rabbits, a recent study compared the incorporation and remodeling processes. Although the bone volume and quality of the grafted area were superior for autogenous bone, the amount of new bone formation after 60 days was similar for autologous and xenogeneic bone blocks [29]. More recently, the healing of collagenated equine bone blocks used as either inlay or onlay for mandibular bone augmentation in rabbits has been assessed [30]. The inlay group showed a faster and higher increase in the percentage of newly formed bone.

Installing implants simultaneously with a bone graft can reduce the total treatment time by eliminating a second surgery. Several clinical [31–36] and experimental [37–41] studies reported data on implants installed with ring grafts secured by the implant for vertical bone augmentation.

To investigate the efficacy of this approach, a randomized clinical trial evaluated marginal bone loss of autogenic bone blocks collected from the chin used for either inlay or onlay grafting with simultaneous implant placement [42]. Bone gain was significantly higher for the inlay group. However, the comparison between xenogeneic bone blocks used for inlay and onlay grafts with implants has not yet been investigated.

Thus, the aim of the present study was to study bone dynamics at inlay and onlay xenografts used for bone augmentation applying a ring technique.

2. Materials and Methods

2.1. Ethical Statements

The Committee on Ethics in the Use of Animals of the Faculty of Dentistry of Ribeirão Preto, University of São Paulo, Brazil approved the experiment on 16 October 2019, as reported in protocol 2019.1.694.58.4. The rules reported in the legislation for animal experimentation in Brazil were strictly followed. The ARRIVE Checklist was used in this study.

2.2. Study Design

This was a split-mouth, prospective, controlled, randomized study. Xenograft blocks were applied to the lateral wall of the mandible using the onlay or inlay techniques. Both blocks were fixed to the recipient sites using an implant. The healing was evaluated after 10 weeks.

2.3. Experimental Animals and Sample Size

Data from a similar study in rabbits were used to determine the sample size [43]. Considering 10% of the difference in the new bone between the two groups as histologically relevant with the maximum standard deviation of 7.4% observed in the study, a sample size of eight animals was obtained to reject the null hypothesis that this response difference is zero by applying $\alpha = 0.05$ and a power of 0.9 (PS, Dupont and Walton D. Plummer). The sample size was increased to 12 to account for possible complications at various levels during the experiment.

Hence, 12 adult male New Zealand White rabbits weighing 3.5–4.0 kg and aged between 5 and 6 months were included in the study. Upon arrival at the institution, animals were properly identified through tags specifying the cage number, species, weight, and scheduled dates for surgery and euthanasia. Additionally, animals received identification numbers on the inner part of the ear using a permanent pen.

2.4. Randomization and Allocation Concealment

An author not involved in animal selection, surgery, and histological evaluation performed the randomization electronically (S.P.X.). The allocation treatment was concealed in opaque sealed envelopes that were opened after recipient site preparation just before the placement of the first xenogeneic block. The histological slides were examined by an assessor (E.F.D.R., see acknowledgements) who was not informed about the allocation treatment. However, the treatment was easily recognized on histological slides.

2.5. Biomaterials

SpBlock is a xenograft block of exclusively collagenated cancellous equine bone (Tecnoss, Giaveno, Italy). This process prevents the ceramization of hydroxyapatite crystals, aiming to accelerate resorption. The blocks were cylindrical with diameters of 7 mm and thicknesses of 3 mm. A hole, in the dimensions of the implant, was prepared in the center of the blocks (Figure 1). The central hole in the blocks was created using a sequence of drills at a speed of 800 rpm and 20 N/m under constant irrigation with 0.9% saline solution until a final diameter of 3.3 mm was obtained, corresponding to the diameter of the implant designated for fixing the blocks.

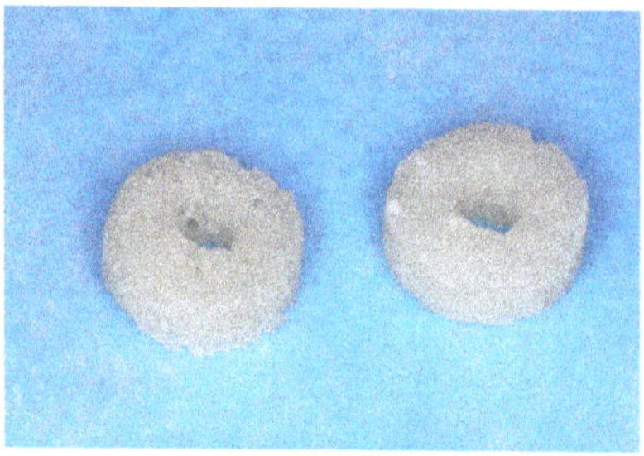

Figure 1. Xenografts with a hole in the center for implant insertion.

Bio-Gide (Geistlich Biomaterials, Wolhusen, LU, Switzerland) is a porcine-derived resorbable membrane composed of types I and III collagen. The bilayer structure contains an outer smooth layer that prevents the invasion of soft tissues and an inner layer that favors the growth of vessels and cells [44].

2.6. Anesthetic Procedures

Anesthetic procedures were carried out using acepromazine (1.0 mg/kg; Acepran, Vetnil, Louveira, São Paulo, Brazil), administered intramuscularly in the hind leg of the animal, and xylazine (3.0 mg/kg; Laboratórios Calier S/A, Barcelona, Spain) combined with ketamine (50.0 mg/kg; União Química Farmacêutica Nacional S/A, Embuguaçú, São Paulo, Brazil), also administered intramuscularly 15 min after the acepromazine administration. Once adequately sedated, the animals underwent prophylactic antibiotic therapy with oxytetracycline (0.2 mL/kg; Biovet, Vargem Grande Paulista, São Paulo, Brazil) administered intramuscularly. Additionally, they received ketoprofen (3.0 mg/kg, 12/12 h, i.m., Ketofen 10%, Merial, Campinas, São Paulo, Brazil) and tramadol hydrochloride 2% (1.0 mg/kg, 12/12 h, subcutaneous, Cronidor, Agener União Saúde Animal, Apucarana, Paraná, Brazil) preoperatively and were maintained postoperatively for the subsequent 3 days.

2.7. Surgical Procedure

One qualified expert surgeon performed all surgeries (V.F.B.; see acknowledgments).

A 2.5–3 mm long incision was made bilaterally on the skin in the lower border of the mandible. The muscles and the periosteum were reflected to expose the lateral surface of the posterior region of the body of the mandible, close to the mandibular angle. At the onlay sites, five calibrated perforations of the cortical layer up to the bone marrow compartment were performed (Figure 2A) using a 1.0 tapered drill (Beavers Jet Burs, Morrisburg, ON, Canada), attached to a straight handpiece, operating at a speed of 20,000 rpm and 20 N/m under constant irrigation with a 0.9% saline solution. This approach was employed to perform five equidistant monocortical perforations, guided by a template crafted from stainless steel. These perforations reached the medullary portion of the recipient site with the purpose of fostering blood and cellular supply to the graft, originating from the endosteal region.

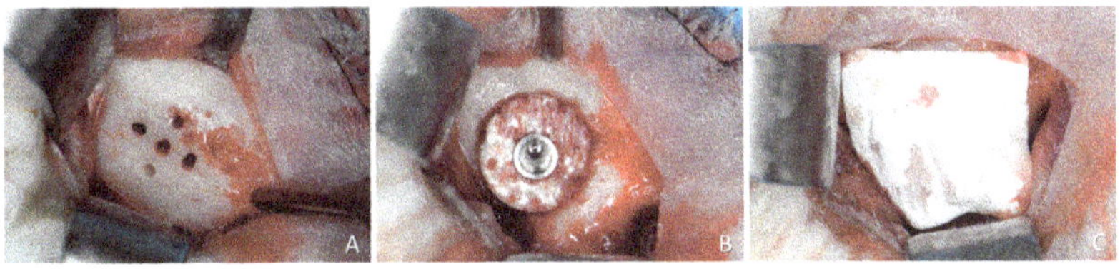

Figure 2. Onlay experimental site. (**A**) Recipient site prepared with perforations. (**B**) Block graft fixed with an implant at the top of the experimental region. (**C**) A collagen membrane placed at the top of the experimental region.

The central perforation was enlarged for implant placement. The xenogeneic bone block was fixed on the prepared region using an implant 8.5 mm long and 3.25 mm in diameter (Leader Medica, Padua, Italy) (Figure 2B). The implant margin was placed at about the level of the graft. A cover screw was positioned on the top of the implant and a collagen membrane was used to cover the experimental region (BioGuide®; Geistlich Pharma AG, Wolhusen, Switzerland) (Figure 2C).

Trephines and drills were used on the opposite side to obtain a defect ~7 mm wide and ~3 mm deep. (Figure 3A). The xenogeneic bone block was adapted within the defect at the level of the adjacent bone and fixed with an implant 8.5 mm long and 3.25 mm in diameter (Leader Medica, Padua, Italy) (Figure 3B). After placement of the cover screw, the region was covered with a collagen membrane (BioGuide®; Geistlich Pharma AG, Wolhusen, Switzerland) (Figure 3C). The wound closure was performed using Vicryl 4-0 (Ethicon, Johnson & Johnson, Cincinnati, OH, USA) for the muscle layers and Nylon 4-0 (Ethicon, Johnson & Johnson, USA) for the skin, employing simple interrupted sutures.

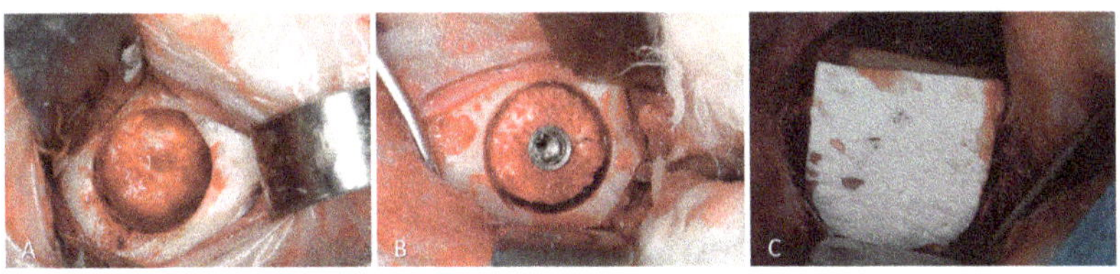

Figure 3. Inlay experimental site. (**A**) Preparation of the 7 mm wide and 3 mm deep defect. (**B**) Placement of the xenograft block inside the defect, secured with an implant. (**C**) Collagen membrane placed on the top of the graft.

2.8. Animal Maintenance

After surgery and during the following 3 days, the animals received ketoprofen (3.0 mg/kg, 12/12 h, i.m., 10% Ketofen, Merial, Campinas, São Paulo, Brazil) and 2% tramadol hydrochloride (1.0 mg/kg 12/12 h, subcutaneous; Cronidor, Agener União Saúde Animal, Apucarana, Paraná, Brazil).

The rabbits were housed in individual metal cages (1 animal/4500 cm^2) in an acclimatized room with split air conditioning, an exhaust fan (27 to 34 air changes/h), and automatic lighting control (12-h light-dark cycle) at the Animal Facility of the Faculty of Dentistry of Ribeirão Preto, University of São Paulo. The animals received dedicated food and had ad libitum access to water. Every day, a careful check of the basic biological functions, feeding and excretion, behavioral signs in relation to postoperative pain, and monitoring of post-surgical infections and surgical wounds for suture care, bleeding, and/or signs of infection was performed.

2.9. Euthanasia

Animals were euthanized by administering an overdose (2.0 mL) of intravenous thiopental 1.0 g (Thiopentax; Cristália, Itapira, São Paulo, Brazil). Euthanasia was conducted in accordance with the guidelines of the Ethics Committee of the Ribeirão Preto School of Dentistry after a 10-week healing period.

2.10. Histological Processing

The experimental regions were dissected, reduced to individual blocks, and fixed in 10% paraformaldehyde for a period of 10 days with regular formaldehyde changes every 2 days. Initially, the specimens were rinsed under running water to ensure complete removal of the fixative agent. Subsequently, they underwent a gradual and ascending dehydration sequence in ethyl alcohol, changed every three days with constant agitation (60%, 80%, 96%, and absolute alcohol twice). Following this, the specimens were immersed in resin (LR WhiteTM HardGrid, London Resin Co., Ltd., Reading, Berkshire, UK) for impregnation, and subsequent polymerization was conducted in an oven at 60 °C.

After polymerization, each block was cut along a transaxial plane at the center of the block, guided by the implant positioned at the center of the graft. Two sections of approximately 100–150 µm were prepared using a precision cutting/grinding instrument (Exakt, Apparatebau, Norderstedt, Germany) and ground until slices with an approximate thickness of 60–80 µm were obtained. The histological sections were stained with Toluidine Blue, Stevenel's Blue, and Alizarin Red.

2.11. Histomorphometric Evaluation

All histomorphometric assessments were performed by an expert assessor (E.F.D.R., see acknowledgements) who did not participate in the other stages of the study, after having compared the results with another expert (D.B.) until inter-rater agreement achieved a Cohen's coefficient of $k > 0.90$.

An Eclipse Ci microscope (Nikon Corporation, Tokyo, Japan) connected to a computer was used for histological assessments by applying a $\times 10$ lens. All histomorphometric assessments were performed with the software NIS Elements D software (v 5.0, Laboratory Imaging, Nikon Corporation, Tokyo, Japan). As a linear evaluation, the distance between the implant margin (M) and the most coronal contact of the bone with the Implant surface (B, coronal level of osseointegration) was measured (Figure 4A,B). The gain of osseointegration was evaluated as the difference between the depth of the original defect (F, 3 mm from M) and the distance M-B. For morphometric measurements, a lattice was superposed on the image by applying point-counting methods. Four regions were evaluated within the grafted region, both sides lateral to the implant: inferior/internal (I-I), inferior/external (I-E), superior/internal (S-I), and superior/external (S-E). The following tissues were assessed: new bone, xenograft, soft tissues (marrow spaces, provisional matrix, dense and loose tissues, and connective tissue), and inflammatory infiltrate (Figure 4A,B). A correlation between the bone percentage in the S-I region and the gain of osseointegration was carried out.

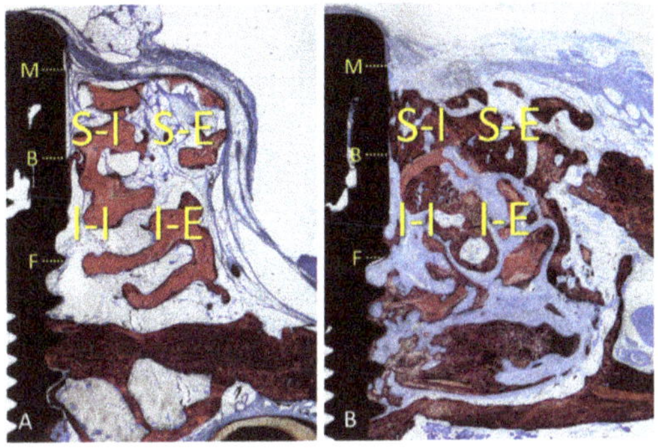

Figure 4. (**A**) Onlay graft; (**B**) inlay graft. Regions evaluated: inferior/internal (I-I), inferior/external (I-E), superior/internal (S-I), and superior/external (S-E). M, implant margin; B, coronal level of osseointegration; F, bottom of the defect.

2.12. Experimental Outcomes and Statistical Methods

Data are reported as the mean ± standard deviation. The primary variables were the mineralized new bone percentage within the grafts and osseointegration gain. The secondary variables were the other tissues evaluated in the morphometric analysis. Differences between onlay and inlay were evaluated using a paired *t*-test or Wilcoxon matched-pairs signed-rank test. The selection of the test was based on the results of normality assessed by applying the Shapiro–Wilk test. GraphPad Prism (version 10.0.2 for Windows, GraphPad Software, Boston, MA, USA) was used for the statistical analysis. The significance level was 5%.

3. Results

3.1. Clinical Outcomes

The healing of the animals was uneventful. All histological slides were available for analysis, with n = 12.

3.2. Descriptive Histological Evaluation

In the onlay group, new bone was found mainly laying on the trabeculae of the xenograft (Figure 5A,B), in some cases reaching the most superficial region (Figure 5C). The areas within the trabeculae were filled with bone marrow in a few cases (Figure 5A,C) or more often by dense soft tissue (Figure 5B).

The configuration of the trabeculae of the graft seemed to have been maintained in several grafts, whereas in other cases, the trabeculae appeared to have lost the original conformation. An inflammatory infiltrate was observed in only one specimen. Most of the implants showed new bone on the surface of the implant within the defect, in some cases up to a distance of <1 mm from the implant margin (Figure 5C).

In the inlay group, new bone lay on the surface of the trabeculae and occupying the spaces among trabeculae (Figure 6A–C). Dense soft tissue was occupying the remaining spaces among the trabeculae. The coronal entrance of the defect was often found closed by new bone formed from the edges of the defect, interconnected with that formed within the graft (Figure 6A–C). The trabeculae of the graft were still present in the region, however, in different proportions in the various specimens. A small inflammatory infiltrate was observed only in one specimen. Most implants showed new bone formed on the implant surface in the defect region, in some cases up to <1 mm from the implant margin (Figure 6A–C).

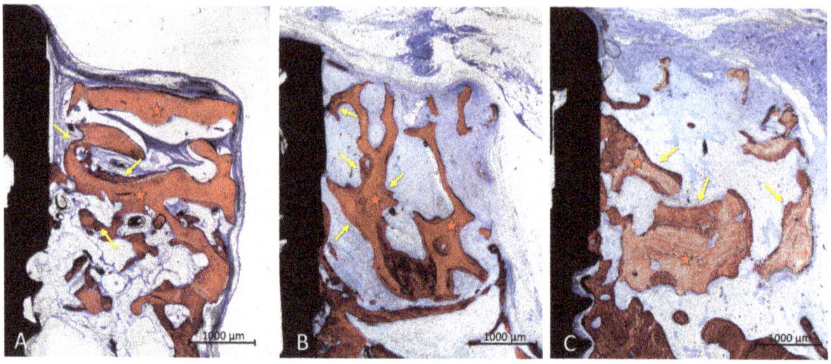

Figure 5. Photomicrographs of ground sections illustrating the healing in the onlay grafts. New bone was mainly found covering the trabeculae (**A**,**B**), in some cases reaching the most coronal regions (**C**). Landmarks indicating examples of tissues: yellow arrows, new bone; red stars, graft. Stevenel's blue and alizarin red stain.

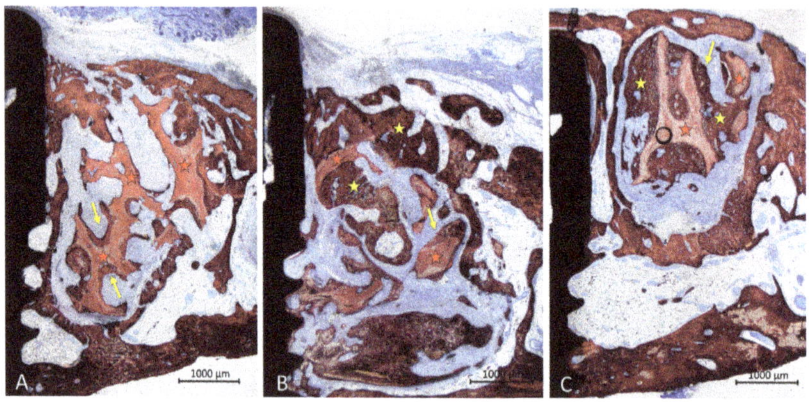

Figure 6. Photomicrographs of ground sections illustrating the healing in the inaly grafts. Bone was found covering the surface of the xenograft but also occupying large spaces within the trabeculae (**A**–**C**). The coronal entrance of the defect was often closed by new bone formed from the margins of the defect and connected by the bone formed within the graft. Landmarks indicating examples of tissues: yellow arrows and stars, new bone; red stars, graft. Stevenel's blue and alizarin red stain.

3.3. Histomorphometric Assessments

After ten weeks of healing, a statistically significantly higher percentage of new bone was found in the inlay compared to the onlay graft, being 19.0 ± 9.3% and 10.4 ± 7.4%, respectively (p = 0.031) (Figure 7).

The new bone percentage was higher at the inlay than at the onlay grafts in all four regions examined, with the difference being statistically significant only for the S-E region. When the bone percentages of the two superior regions were merged (mean S-E and S-I), a statistically significant difference was found between the two groups (p = 0.010).

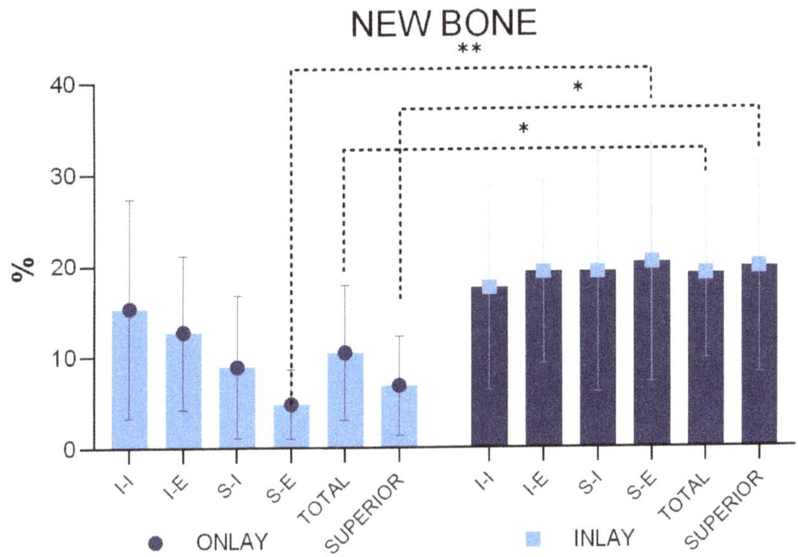

Figure 7. New bone percentages in the various regions examined. * $p < 0.05$; ** $p < 0.01$ (Graphs produced with GraphPad Prism).

The mean percentage of the xenograft did not yield statistically significant differences in any of the regions evaluated. An inflammatory infiltrate was observed only in one specimen of the onlay graft (Figure 8).

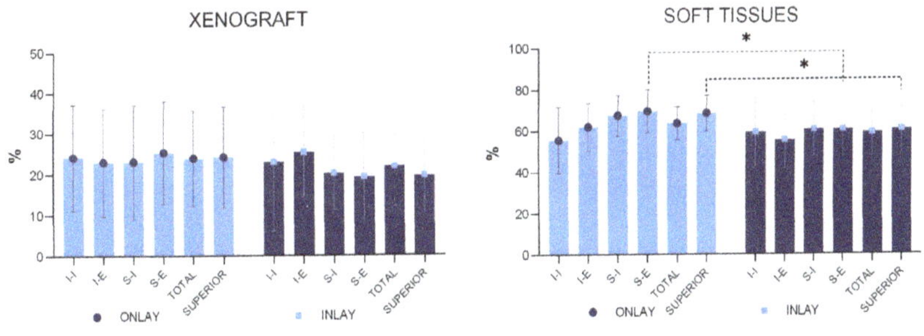

Figure 8. Xenograft and soft tissue percentages in the various regions examined. * $p < 0.05$ (Graphs produced with GraphPad Prism).

Even though, in some cases, the coronal level of osseointegration on the implant was located <1 mm from the implant margin, other sites presented any or very little bone gain on the implant surface above the 3 mm deep original defect. The mean gains were 0.95 ± 1.05% in the onlay group and 0.78 ± 0.71% in the inlay group ($p = 0.603$). The r-value correlation between the new bone percentage in the superior interior region S-I and the level of osseointegration was 0.7 (a strong positive linear relationship).

4. Discussion

The current research focused on comparing the bone dynamics of implants installed with inlay or onlay grafts for lateral bone augmentation in the mandible of rabbits. The results demonstrated a higher new bone mean percentage in the inlay graft (19.0 ± 9.3%) compared to the onlay graft (10.4 ± 7.4%; $p = 0.031$). The highest differences in bone formation between the two groups were observed in the region closer to the top of the grafts, i.e., the furthest regions from the bone walls.

The reasons for these differences in the proportion of new bone are to be referred to the different characteristics of the recipient regions. Indeed, inlay grafts were inserted into self-contained defects presenting walls at the base and around the graft. This means that the grafts could rely on bone production from various sources located around them. Instead, the onlay grafts could only rely on bone formed from the cortical layer in contact with the base of the graft. From that recipient site, the new bone had to grow toward the top and the lateral sides of the graft.

In the onlay group, aiming to favor new bone formation, several perforations of the cortical layer were made, reaching the marrow spaces. This procedure has been shown to improve the healing within the graft. In a study on rabbits, the lateral aspect of the mandible angle was prepared with perforations only on one side, while the opposite side was left intact [45]. Block grafts obtained from the iliac crest were secured on the mandibular recipient sites. Revascularization, volume/density maintenance, and the occurrence of bone remodeling proteins were evaluated for different periods of healing. A higher loss of volume was observed in the intact site graft while a higher bone density was measured in the perforated sites. The VEGF labeling became apparent already after 3 days in the perforated group while, in the intact sites, the labeling became evident after 5 days, exhibiting an earlier angiogenesis rate in the former than in the latter groups. The immuno-labeling of osteoblastic lineage showed an accelerated bone remodeling process in the perforated sites. The effect of these perforations was illustrated in detail in another study in which grafts collected from the calvaria were applied on the mandibular angle prepared with perforations [46].

The onlay graft can only count on the osteoconductivity of the biomaterial, which is of foremost importance. Indeed, considering the results from experimental studies, the lack of osteoconductivity of the biomaterial might lead to failures. In a dog study, block grafts composed of deproteinized bovine bone material (DBBM) were placed as onlay on the lateral wall of the alveolar bone in the mandible. A minimal incorporation of the xenograft was observed, limited to the base close to the recipient site [47]. In another experiment in dogs [48], similar DBBM blocks were placed as inlay grafts in defects prepared in the alveolar bone crest in the mandible. On the opposite side of the mandible, an autogenous bone block was used as a graft. While the autogenous bone block presented a perfect incorporation to the recipient site, the xenograft failed to be incorporated, showing, in most cases, a layer of connective tissue interposed between the graft and the recipient sites. Instead, when collagenated blocks were used, new bone was formed within the graft, laying on the trabeculae of the xenograft and reaching the furthest regions from the recipient site [43].

The superior outcome in bone growth of the inlay compared to the onlay block grafts could be related to the positioning of the graft within a self-contained defect that, being delimited by bone walls, offered multiple sources for bone growth. Depending on the dimensions, self-contained defects have the potential to heal spontaneously, similar to the extraction sockets. The spontaneous healing of critical-sized defects was evaluated in rabbits in both the calvaria and mandible [49]. In each animal, through-and-through circumferential defects were prepared, 10 mm in diameter in the calvaria and 11 mm in diameter in the mandible. Autogenous bone or biphasic calcium phosphate granules were placed on the defects of one side of the mandible to fill them out, and the opposite defects were left to heal spontaneously. Both microCT and histological analysis revealed a failure in the closure of the empty defects. The defect applied in the present study presented more favorable conditions compared to the study mentioned above, i.e., smaller dimensions and a box conformation that also allowed bone formation from the base of the defect.

In another experimental study on rabbits [50], 2- to 3-mm-deep box defects of different dimensions (4, 5, 6, 8, and 10 mm) were prepared in the mandible. After 12 weeks of healing, the smallest defects were closed with newly formed bone. However, the 8-mm-

and 10-mm-wide defects persisted underfilled. The defects applied in the present study had a box conformation and a diameter of 7 mm. Under such conditions, it is reasonable to assume that a certain degree of spontaneous healing should be expected.

However, an implant was placed in the center of the defect to fix the graft. This implant affected the total volume of the defect and eventually transformed a 7 mm critical-sized defect into a circumferential peri-implant marginal defect with a gap of <2 mm. This allows us to suppose that the placement of an implant might accelerate the healing. In contrast, it has been already demonstrated that the implant delays the healing of marginal defects [51]. In fact, in a marginal defect around an implant, new bone is formed from the lateral walls towards the implant surface and it stops approximately 0.4 mm from the surface, leaving a residual narrow defect around the implant surface, occupied by connective tissues. This defect is closed over time by newly formed bone only if the surface has osteoconductive properties [52]. If the implant surface is not osteoconductive, the residual narrow defect will be not filled by new bone [52,53]. In the present study, an incomplete mean gain of implant osseointegration within the graft region was observed in both the inlay (0.78 mm) and onlay (0.95 mm) groups. In several cases, the osseointegration reached a distance of <1 mm from the implant margin in both groups, showing good osteoconductive properties of the implant surface. The low mean gain of osseointegration is due to a large variability of the results, the reasons for which could be attributed to an insufficient new bone content in the internal regions of some grafts, especially in the superior-internal region. In the absence of bone close to the implant surface, the gain in osseointegration is hampered. This assumption is substantiated by the strong positive linear correlation between osseointegration gain and the percentage of new bone in the superior-internal region.

In another comparable experiment on rabbits, a similar pattern of bone formation was observed as in the present study [30]. In that study, the onlay and inlay xenografts were of the same nature as those used in the present study. However, the grafts were secured on the recipient sites with a fixation screw. Two periods of healing were analyzed, i.e., 2 and 10 weeks. The results showed a higher percentage of new bone at the inlay compared to the onlay grafts. The percentage of the xenograft decreased by approximately one-third between the two periods of healing. In the present study, the evaluation was performed after only 10 weeks of healing. However, with the percentage of the residual grafts after 10 weeks being similar between the two studies, it might be supposed that a similar percentage of graft resorption occurred in both studies.

In the present study, complete closure of the coronal entrance of the defects was observed in several specimens of the inlay blocks. This agrees with similar observations reported in the study mentioned above [30].

The present study adopted a "ring" technique with immediate implant installation. This technique was used for vertical augmentation, the results of which have been reported in systematic reviews of both clinical [54] and animal [55] studies.

The animal model used is a limitation of the present study so the data should be interpreted with caution. Several limitations of the study should be considered, such as the faster rate of healing in rabbits compared to humans, as shown for implant osseointegration [56]. Moreover, the healing of critical defects in the body and the angle of the mandible is hampered by the growth of soft tissue in the region [57] and limited blood supply [58]. These conditions might have compromised healing.

Nevertheless, the experimental studies only reveal possible outcomes that should be considered when similar procedures are applied in humans, and eventually confirmed or refuted. Longer periods of healing should be analyzed.

5. Conclusions

The inlay grafts exhibited a higher new bone percentage than the onlay block grafts possibly due to the defect conformation that presented more sources for bone formation. The trabecular conformation and the composition of the grafts made possible the expression of the osteoconductive properties of the material used. This resulted, in several specimens, in the growth of bone toward the most superior regions in both grafts and in the closure of the coronal entrance of the defects in the inlay group. The clinical relevance of this experiment is that the ring technique applied as an inlay method could be suitable for bone augmentation. However, in clinical practice, a vertical defect rarely presents conditions that allow for performing a purely inlay technique. In the best conditions, an intermediate situation between inlay and onlay can be encountered. It is therefore important to model the recipient region in a way that brings this region as close as possible to a self-contained defect. Some xenograft blocks have been shown to have poor osteoconductive properties, making graft selection of critical importance. Furthermore, even if the xenografts have the same conformation as spongy bone, it is necessary for these pseudo-bony trabeculae to be reabsorbed to make room for newly formed bone trabeculae. Simply forming bone on the surface of the xeno-trabeculae cannot be considered optimal healing. This, in turn, means that further studies applying grafts of different materials and conformations are needed to improve outcomes, especially when the grafts are used as onlay.

Author Contributions: Conceptualization, N.K., S.P.X., K.M. and D.B.; methodology, N.K., S.P.X. and D.B.; validation, K.M., Y.N. and S.B.; formal analysis, N.K., E.R.S. and D.B.; investigation, S.P.X. and E.R.S.; resources, S.P.X., D.B. and Y.N.; data curation, N.K. and D.B.; writing—original draft preparation, N.K., E.R.S. and D.B; writing—review and editing, N.K., S.P.X., D.B. and S.B.; visualization, K.M. and Y.N.; supervision, S.P.X., D.B. and S.B.; project administration, S.P.X., D.B. and Y.N.; funding acquisition, D.B. and Y.N. All authors have read and agreed to the published version of the manuscript.

Funding: The experiment was financially supported by the ARDEC Academy, Rimini, Italy.

Institutional Review Board Statement: This research project was approved by the Committee on Ethics in the Use of Animals of the Faculty of Dentistry of Ribeirão Preto, University of São Paulo, Brazil, on 16 October 2019, protocol #2019.1.694.58.4.

Informed Consent Statement: Not applicable.

Data Availability Statement: The data are available following a reasonable request.

Acknowledgments: We thank Vitor Ferreira Balan for the surgical procedures and Sebastiao Blanco (University of São Paulo, Faculty of Dentistry of Ribeirão Preto) for processing the histological slides. The scientific contribution in the histological assessment by Ermenegildo Federico De Rossi (ARDEC Academy, Italy) is greatly appreciated.

Conflicts of Interest: The authors declare no conflict of interest.

References

1. Felice, P.; Marchetti, C.; Piattelli, A.; Pellegrino, G.; Checchi, V.; Worthington, H.; Esposito, M. Vertical ridge augmentation of the atrophic posterior mandible with interpositional block grafts: Bone from the iliac crest versus bovine anorganic bone. *Eur. J. Oral. Implantol.* **2008**, *1*, 183–198.
2. Cordaro, L.; Amadé, D.S.; Cordaro, M. Clinical results of alveolar ridge augmentation with mandibular block bone grafts in partially edentulous patients prior to implant placement. *Clin. Oral Implant. Res.* **2002**, *13*, 103–111. [CrossRef]
3. Chiapasco, M.; Zaniboni, M.; Rimondini, L. Autogenous onlay bone grafts vs. alveolar distraction osteogenesis for the correction of vertically deficient edentulous ridges: A 2–4-year prospective study on humans. *Clin. Oral. Implant. Res.* **2007**, *18*, 432–440. [CrossRef]
4. Marx, R.E. Bone and bone graft healing. *Oral. Maxillofac. Surg. Clin. N. Am.* **2007**, *19*, 455–466. [CrossRef]
5. Habal, M.B. Bone grafting in craniofacial surgery. *Clin. Plast. Surg.* **1994**, *21*, 349–363. [CrossRef]
6. Louis, P.J.; Sittitavornwong, S. Managing Bone Grafts for the Mandible. *Oral Maxillofac. Surg. Clin. N. Am.* **2019**, *31*, 317–330. [CrossRef] [PubMed]
7. Stellingsma, C.; Raghoebar, G.M.; Meijer, H.J.; Batenburg, R.H. Reconstruction of the extremely resorbed mandible with interposed bone grafts and placement of endosseous implants. A preliminary report on outcome of treatment and patients' satisfaction. *Br. J. Oral Maxillofac. Surg.* **1998**, *36*, 290–295. [CrossRef] [PubMed]

8. Choi, B.H.; Lee, S.H.; Huh, J.Y.; Han, S.G. Use of the sandwich osteotomy plus an interpositional allograft for vertical augmentation of the alveolar ridge. *J. Craniomaxillofac. Surg.* **2004**, *32*, 51–54. [CrossRef] [PubMed]
9. Stoelinga, P.J.; Blijdorp, P.A.; Ross, R.R.; De Koomen, H.A.; Huybers, T.J. Augmentation of the atrophic mandible with interposed bone grafts and particulate hydroxylapatite. *J. Oral Maxillofac. Surg.* **1986**, *44*, 353–360. [CrossRef] [PubMed]
10. Yeung, R. Surgical management of the partially edentulous atrophic mandibular ridge using a modified sandwich osteotomy: A case report. *Int. J. Oral Maxillofac. Implant.* **2005**, *20*, 799–803.
11. Jensen, O.T. Alveolar segmental "sandwich" osteotomies for posterior edentulous mandibular sites for dental implants. *J. Oral Maxillofac. Surg.* **2006**, *64*, 471–475. [CrossRef]
12. Marchetti, C.; Trasarti, S.; Corinaldesi, G.; Felice, P. Interpositional bone grafts in the posterior mandibular region: A report on six patients. *Int. J. Periodontics Restor. Dent.* **2007**, *27*, 547–555.
13. Bianchi, A.; Felice, P.; Lizio, G.; Marchetti, C. Alveolar distraction osteogenesis versus inlay bone grafting in posterior mandibular atrophy: A prospective study. *Oral Surg. Oral Med. Oral Pathol. Oral Radiol. Endod.* **2008**, *105*, 282–292. [CrossRef]
14. Schwartz-Arad, D.; Levin, L.; Sigal, L. Surgical success of intraoral autogenous block onlay bone grafting for alveolar ridge augmentation. *Implant. Dent.* **2005**, *14*, 131–138. [CrossRef]
15. Felice, P.; Pistilli, R.; Lizio, G.; Pellegrino, G.; Nisii, A.; Marchetti, C. Inlay versus onlay iliac bone grafting in atrophic posterior mandible: A prospective controlled clinical trial for the comparison of two techniques. *Clin. Implant. Dent. Relat. Res.* **2009**, *11* (Suppl. 1), e69–e82. [CrossRef]
16. Donovan, M.G.; Dickerson, N.C.; Mitchell, J.C. Calvarial bone harvest and grafting techniques for maxillary and mandibular implant surgery. *Atlas. Oral Maxillofac. Surg. Clin. N. Am.* **1994**, *2*, 109–122. [CrossRef]
17. Von Arx, T.; Cochran, D.L.; Hermann, J.S.; Schenk, R.K.; Higginbottom, F.L.; Buser, D. Lateral ridge augmentation and implant placement: An experimental study evaluating implant osseointegration in different augmentation materials in the canine mandible. *Int. J. Oral Maxillofac. Implants.* **2001**, *16*, 343–354. [PubMed]
18. Chiriac, G.; Herten, M.; Schwarz, F.; Rothamel, D.; Becker, J. Autogenous bone chips: Influence of a new piezoelectric device (Piezosurgery) on chip morphology, cell viability and differentiation. *J. Clin. Periodontol.* **2005**, *32*, 994–999. [CrossRef] [PubMed]
19. Nowzari, H.; Aalam, A.A. Mandibular cortical bone graft part 2: Surgical technique, applications, and morbidity. *Compend. Contin. Educ. Dent.* **2007**, *28*, 274–280, quiz 281–282. [PubMed]
20. Clavero, J.; Lundgren, S. Ramus or chin grafts for maxillary sinus inlay and local onlay augmentation: Comparison of donor site morbidity and complications. *Clin. Implant. Dent. Relat. Res.* **2003**, *5*, 154–160. [CrossRef] [PubMed]
21. Chiapasco, M.; Zaniboni, M.; Boisco, M. Augmentation procedures for the rehabilitation of deficient edentulous ridges with oral implants. *Clin. Oral Implant. Res.* **2006**, *17* (Suppl. 2), 136–159. [CrossRef]
22. Nkenke, E.; Schultze-Mosgau, S.; Radespiel-Tröger, M.; Kloss, F.; Neukam, F.W. Morbidity of harvesting of chin grafts: A prospective study. *Clin. Oral Implant. Res.* **2001**, *12*, 495–502. [CrossRef] [PubMed]
23. Nkenke, E.; Weisbach, V.; Winckler, E.; Kessler, P.; Schultze-Mosgau, S.; Wiltfang, J.; Neukam, F.W. Morbidity of harvesting of bone grafts from the iliac crest for preprosthetic augmentation procedures: A prospective study. *Int. J. Oral Maxillofac. Surg.* **2004**, *33*, 157–163. [CrossRef] [PubMed]
24. Von Arx, T.; Häfliger, J.; Chappuis, V. Neurosensory disturbances following bone harvesting in the symphysis: A prospective clinical study. *Clin. Oral Implant. Res.* **2005**, *16*, 432–439. [CrossRef] [PubMed]
25. McAllister, B.S.; Haghighat, K. Bone augmentation techniques. *J. Periodontol.* **2007**, *78*, 377–396. [CrossRef] [PubMed]
26. Pistilli, R.; Felice, P.; Piatelli, M.; Nisii, A.; Barausse, C.; Esposito, M. Blocks of autogenous bone versus xenografts for the rehabilitation of atrophic jaws with dental implants: Preliminary data from a pilot randomized controlled trial. *Eur. J. Oral Implantol.* **2014**, *7*, 153–171.
27. Al Ruhaimi, K.A. Bone graft substitutes: A comparative qualitative histologic review of current osteoconductive grafting materials. *Int. J. Oral Maxillofac. Implant.* **2001**, *16*, 105–114.
28. Troeltzsch, M.; Troeltzsch, M.; Kauffmann, P.; Gruber, R.; Brockmeyer, P.; Moser, N.; Rau, A.; Schliephake, H. Clinical efficacy of grafting materials in alveolar ridge augmentation: A systematic review. *J. Craniomaxillofac. Surg.* **2016**, *44*, 1618–1629. [CrossRef]
29. Silva, E.R.; Balan, V.F.; Botticelli, D.; Soldini, C.; Okamoto, R.; Xavier, S.P. Histomorphometric, Immunohistochemical and Microtomographic Comparison between Autogenous and Xenogenous Bone Blocks for Mandibular Lateral Augmentation in Rabbits. *Materials* **2021**, *14*, 6049. [CrossRef]
30. Sakaguchi, R.; Xavier, S.P.; Morinaga, K.; Botticelli, D.; Silva, E.R.; Nakajima, Y.; Baba, S. Healing of Collagenated Cancellous Equine Bone Blocks Used as Inlay or Onlay for Lateral Bone Augmentation in Rabbits. *Preprints* **2023**, 2023090756. [CrossRef]
31. Peñarrocha-Diago, M.; Gómez-Adrián, M.D.; García-Mira, B.; Ivorra-Sais, M. Bone grafting simultaneous to implant placement. Present of a case. *Med. Oral Patol. Oral Cir. Bucal.* **2005**, *10*, 444–447. [PubMed]
32. Omara, M.; Abdelwahed, N.; Ahmed, M.; Hindy, M. Simultaneous implant placement with ridge augmentation using an autogenous bone ring transplant. *Int. J. Oral Maxillofac. Surg.* **2016**, *45*, 535–544. [CrossRef]
33. Yuce, M.O.; Adali, E.; Turk, G.; Isik, G.; Gunbay, T. Three-dimensional bone grafting in dental implantology using autogenous bone ring transplant: Clinical outcomes of a one-stage technique. *Niger. J. Clin. Pract.* **2019**, *22*, 977–981. [CrossRef]

34. Chandra, R.V.; Shivateja, K.; Reddy, A.A. Autogenous Bone Ring Transplant vs Autologous Growth Factor-Enriched Bone Graft Matrix in Extraction Sockets With Deficient Buccal Bone: A Comparative Clinical Study. *Int. J. Oral Maxillofac. Implant.* **2019**, *34*, 1424–1433. [CrossRef] [PubMed]
35. Giraddi, G.B.; Saifi, A.M. Bone Ring Augmentation Around Immediate Implants: A Clinical and Radiographic Study. *Ann. Maxillofac. Surg.* **2017**, *7*, 92–97. [PubMed]
36. Wychowanski, P.; Woliński, J.; Morawiec, T.; Kownacki, P.; Starzynska, A.; Kosieradzki, M.; Fiedor, P. Preliminary Clinical Data and the Comparison of the Safety and Efficacy of Autogenous Bone Grafts Versus Xenograft Implantations in Vertical Bone Deficiencies Before Dental Implant Installation. *Transpl. Proc.* **2020**, *52*, 2248–2251. [CrossRef]
37. Benlidayi, M.E.; Tatli, U.; Salimov, F.; Tükel, H.C.; Yuksel, O. Comparison of autogenous and allograft bone rings in surgically created vertical bone defects around implants in a sheep model. *Clin. Oral Implant. Res.* **2018**, *29*, 1155–1162. [CrossRef]
38. Jinno, Y.; Jimbo, R.; Lindstrom, M.; Sawase, T.; Lilin, T.; Becktor, J.P. Vertical bone augmentation using ring technique with three different materials in the sheep mandible bone. *Int. J. Oral Maxillofac. Implant.* **2018**, *33*, 1057–1063. [CrossRef]
39. Haga-Tsujimura, M.; Nakahara, K.; Kobayashi, E.; Igarashi, K.; Schaller, B.; Saulacic, N. Single-staged implant placement using bone ring technique with and without membrane placement: An experimental study in the beagle dog. *Clin. Oral Implant. Res.* **2018**, *29*, 263–276. [CrossRef]
40. Nakahara, K.; Haga-Tsujimura, M.; Sawada, K.; Kobayashi, E.; Mottini, M.; Schaller, B.; Saulacic, N. Single-staged vs. two-staged implant placement using bone ring technique in vertically deficient alveolar ridges—Part 1: Histomorphometric and micro-CT analysis. *Clin. Oral Implant. Res.* **2016**, *27*, 1384–1391. [CrossRef]
41. Nakahara, K.; Haga-Tsujimura, M.; Sawada, K.; Kobayashi, E.; Schaller, B.; Saulacic, N. Single-staged vs. two-staged implant placement in vertically deficient alveolar ridges using bone ring technique—Part 2: Implant osseointegration. *Clin. Oral Implant. Res.* **2017**, *28*, e31–e38. [CrossRef]
42. El Zahwy, M.; Taha, S.A.A.K.; Mounir, R.; Mounir, M. Assessment of vertical ridge augmentation and marginal bone loss using autogenous onlay vs inlay grafting techniques with simultaneous implant placement in the anterior maxillary esthetic zone: A randomized clinical trial. *Clin. Implant. Dent. Relat. Res.* **2019**, *21*, 1140–1147. [CrossRef] [PubMed]
43. Kanayama, M.; Botticelli, D.; Apaza Alccayhuaman, K.A.; Yonezawa, D.; Silva, E.R.; Xavier, S.P. The Impact on the Healing of Bioactivation with Argon Plasma of a Xenogeneic Graft with Adequate Fixation but Poor Adaptation to the Recipient Site: An Experimental Study in Rabbits. *Int. J. Oral Maxillofac. Implant.* **2021**, *36*, 703–714. [CrossRef] [PubMed]
44. Schwarz, F.; Sager, M.; Ferrari, D.; Mihatovic, I.; Becker, J. Influence of recombinant human platelet-derived growth factor on lateral ridge augmentation using biphasic calcium phosphate and guided bone regeneration: A histomorphometric study in dogs. *J. Periodontol.* **2009**, *80*, 1315–1323. [CrossRef]
45. Faria, P.E.; Okamoto, R.; Bonilha-Neto, R.M.; Xavier, S.P.; Santos, A.C.; Salata, L.A. Immunohistochemical, tomographic and histological study on onlay iliac grafts remodeling. *Clin. Oral Implant. Res.* **2008**, *19*, 393–401. [CrossRef] [PubMed]
46. Caneva, M.; Botticelli, D.; Carneiro Martins, E.N.; Caneva, M.; Lang, N.P.; Xavier, S.P. Healing at the interface between recipient sites and autologous block bone grafts affixed by either position or lag screw methods: A histomorphometric study in rabbits. *Clin. Oral Implant. Res.* **2017**, *28*, 1484–1491. [CrossRef]
47. Araújo, M.G.; Sonohara, M.; Hayacibara, R.; Cardaropoli, G.; Lindhe, J. Lateral ridge augmentation by the use of grafts comprised of autologous bone or a biomaterial. An experiment in the dog. *J. Clin. Periodontol.* **2002**, *29*, 1122–1131. [CrossRef] [PubMed]
48. De Santis, E.; Lang, N.P.; Favero, G.; Beolchini, M.; Morelli, F.; Botticelli, D. Healing at mandibular block-grafted sites. An experimental study in dogs. *Clin. Oral Implant. Res.* **2015**, *26*, 516–522. [CrossRef]
49. Kotagudda Ranganath, S.; Schlund, M.; Delattre, J.; Ferri, J.; Chai, F. Bilateral double site (calvarial and mandibular) critical-size bone defect model in rabbits for evaluation of a craniofacial tissue engineering constructs. *Mater Today Bio.* **2022**, *14*, 100267. [CrossRef]
50. Wang, Y.; Zhang, X.; Mei, S.; Li, Y.; Khan, A.A.; Guan, S.; Li, X. Determination of critical-sized defect of mandible in a rabbit model: Micro-computed tomography, and histological evaluation. *Heliyon* **2023**, *9*, e18047. [CrossRef]
51. Botticelli, D.; Berglundh, T.; Buser, D.; Lindhe, J. Appositional bone formation in marginal defects at implants. *Clin. Oral Implant. Res.* **2003**, *14*, 1–9. [CrossRef] [PubMed]
52. Botticelli, D.; Berglundh, T.; Lindhe, J. Resolution of bone defects of varying dimension and configuration in the marginal portion of the peri-implant bone. An experimental study in the dog. *J. Clin. Periodontol.* **2004**, *31*, 309–317. [CrossRef] [PubMed]
53. Akimoto, K.; Becker, W.; Persson, R.; Baker, D.A.; Rohrer, M.D.; O'Neal, R.B. Evaluation of titanium implants placed into simulated extraction sockets: A study in dogs. *Int. J. Oral Maxillofac. Implant.* **1999**, *14*, 351–360.
54. Sáez-Alcaide, L.M.; Brinkmann, J.C.; Sánchez-Labrador, L.; Pérez-González, F.; Molinero-Mourelle, P.; López-Quiles, J. Effectiveness of the bone ring technique and simultaneous implant placement for vertical ridge augmentation: A systematic review. *Int. J. Implant. Dent.* **2020**, *6*, 82. [CrossRef]
55. Gaikwad, A.M.; Joshi, A.A.; Padhye, A.M.; Nadgere, J.B. Autogenous bone ring for vertical bone augmentation procedure with simultaneous implant placement: A systematic review of histologic and histomorphometric outcomes in animal studies. *J. Prosthet. Dent.* **2021**, *126*, 626–635. [CrossRef]
56. Botticelli, D.; Lang, N.P. Dynamics of osseointegration in various human and animal models—A comparative analysis. *Clin. Oral Implant. Res.* **2017**, *28*, 742–748. [CrossRef]

57. Herford, A.S.; Boyne, P.J. Reconstruction of mandibular continuity defects with bone morphogenetic protein-2 (rhBMP-2). *J. Oral Maxillofac. Surg.* **2008**, *66*, 616–624. [CrossRef]
58. Chim, H.; Gosain, A.K. Biomaterials in craniofacial surgery: Experimental studies and clinical application. *J. Craniofac. Surg.* **2009**, *20*, 29–33. [CrossRef]

MDPI AG
Grosspeteranlage 5
4052 Basel
Switzerland
Tel.: +41 61 683 77 34

Materials Editorial Office
E-mail: materials@mdpi.com
www.mdpi.com/journal/materials

www.ingramcontent.com/pod-product-compliance
Lightning Source LLC
Chambersburg PA
CBHW041953260926
51850CB00019B/2681
9783725865543